A Heart Like Mine

Finding God's Will for Your Life

By Cindy Valenti-Scinto

Adelphos Books
Spokane Valley, Washington

A Heart Like Mine

by Cindy Valenti-Scinto

www.AHeartLikeMine.com

Published by: Adelphos Books
18401 E. 8th Ave. Ste. 102
Spokane Valley, WA 99016
www.AHeartLikeMine.com

Cover design and artwork by Linda Schneider
Author photo on back taken by Photographic Designs, Rock Hill, SC, www.pennyyoung.com

First Printing, August 2008
Printed in the United States of America

ISBN: 978-0-615-23883-8

Dedication

This book is dedicated to my heart donor Danielle—my "*Angel on Earth*." Although I never knew you face-to-face, I know your very essence. Each time your heart beats in my chest, I am reminded of the life you gave so that I could live.

Greater love has no one than this,
than to lay down one's life for his friends.
John 15:13

4-28-2009
Dear Linda,
Be blessed this day!
May your heart be touched!
Cindy

Table of Contents

Acknowledgements

First of all, my husband John deserves the utmost recognition for his unwavering dedication to holding up the proclamation, "in sickness and health" as he takes care of me day after day, never stopping to complain once. I would not be here without his love, faithful help, encouragement, wisdom, and support. I love you.

And my son Jonathan, you had to persevere through entering your teen years worrying your mom may not be alive when you came home from school each day. Much was delayed or missed due to my constant illness. I love you for being a caring, loving, son who always found a way to cheer me up. I will never forget the first time I was in the ICU unit and you had your Dad read Psalm 86 to me. You thought I would like how it spoke of God fighting for us and helping the needy. You are the best son anyone could *grow up with*!

The countless friends and people, some I don't even know, who did so much for me—there aren't enough pages for all of you. The closest ones who sacrificed much are dear to my heart: John, Terry, Misty, and Cody Craig, Dave and Angie Nerren, Josh Nerren, Royce and Susan Hershberger, Chris and Linda Schneider, Jeff Kuntz, Kelly Henssler, Michelle, Darin, and Felicia Vierth, Joel and Beverley Novin, the ladies from The Alter church, and the ladies from Valley Fourth Memorial Church.

There were Pastors and their wives who stood by us in deed and prayer: Pastor Ray and Bertha Duran, Pastor John and Carolyn Underhill, The elders from Valley Fourth Memorial Church, Pastor John and Shaunna Higgins, Pastor David and Tot Landry, Pastor Tim and Penny Tyler, and Pastor Rick and Dianne Kahlbau.

The doctors and staff my life depended on and still does—I can never find a way to properly thank you all: Special thanks to Dr. Canaday for believing in me and never using the word "psychology," Dr. Chilson, Dr. Icenogle. Dr. Sandler, Dr. Sestero, Sacred Heart Medical Center staff, the nurses on 6-South and 6-North, ICU nurses, Carole Fenkner from Blue Cross Blue Shield, Dr. Stegmann, Dr. Boehmer, the staff at the cath lab in Sacred Heart—especially dear, sweet "Carol," and big, bad "Dave," the staff of Spokane Cardiovascular Services, the paramedics with American Medical Response and the ER nurses at Sacred Heart Medical Center who were there to usher me back to earth!

The staff at The King's *High* Way who always pray, encourage, and put up with me! Pastor Tim, Nancy, Debbie, Kathryn, Davey, Meshell, and Lori: You are my "base camp" whenever a new mountain gets in my way! And others I know from the ministry who always support me: Chuck, Robin, Marilyn, Nancy, Liz, Melanie, Al, Rene, Angel, the Tuesday night Bible Study at Koinonia House, and the ladies from the Calvary Chapel Coeur d'Alene, Bible Study: Beve, Barby, Barbara, Carol, Dianne, Rene, Helen, Dottie, Joyce,

My family has always prayed for me and supported John, Jonathan, and I: My Mom and Pete, Charlie (who went to be with the Lord) and Sari, Steve and Jian, Annie and Gerry, Nanette and Bill, Lori, My mother-in-law Rose, Joe and Lynn, Paul, Tom, Rich and Melanie, and many other family members both here and abroad in Italy.

My heartfelt thanks, admiration, and appreciation go to Donna Goodrich for her incredible proofreading skills. But more importantly, Donna, you are my friend, mentor, and a Godly woman who has taught me much.

In memory are my Dad, Joseph Valenti, who always encouraged me to write and my brother Charlie who was *there for me when I needed him*.

Charlotte, Danielle's Mom—you have provided the completion for this book. I love you.

Thank you, God, for allowing all these people to have a hand in my life. You, my Father in Heaven, started this journey and You will bring it to completion, in Your time.

Foreword

With over 30 years as Senior Pastor of a large church, and as many years serving as Chaplain for the local Fire Department, I regularly encounter people faced with a variety of challenging situations. Few I have dealt with have been tested as dramatically and severely as Cindy Valenti-Scinto and her family.

The impact of Cindy's story is not to be found only in the life and death struggle of her failing physical heart and related medical difficulties. The penetrating power of this book is revealed in the testimony of her spiritual discoveries. It is the development of a spiritual heart—a heart that by faith has learned to rest in a God who proves Himself real in the unexpected storms of everyday life.

> *I praise you because I am fearfully and wonderfully made; your works are wonderful, I know that full well. My frame was not hidden from you when I was made in the secret place. When I was woven together in the depths of the earth, your eyes saw my unformed body. All the days ordained for me were written in your book before one of them came to be* (Psalm 139:14-16 NIV).

The Hebrew word for "ordained" means to form, fashion, shape, or frame human activity. It is to plan or purpose a situation. It relates to something or someone being predetermined or formed according to a divine plan and purpose. Biblically it is often used of potters who form their creations.

A Heart Like Mine is the experience of young wife and mother as she learns to embrace her days as *ordained* by God. Cindy's unforeseen and seemingly never ending physical trials have turned her world upside down. This is a thought provoking account of a journey in understanding God's will for our lives in the midst of extreme difficulties.

Through the Word of God and prayer, Cindy has gleaned timeless truths about a God who can be trusted even when our own hearts prove to be broken and flawed. This is a revealing portrait of each of our lives to one extent or another. It is a compelling call to recognize the human heart as fatally spoiled by sin. This book challenges readers to seek remedy in Jesus Christ and the spiritual transplant He alone can provide.

Biblically sound and well researched, Cindy writes *A Heart Like Mine* for every person who has every wondered *why bad things happen to good people.*

Dr. Robert V. Smith
Senior Pastor, Mt. Spokane Church
Spokane, Washington
Chaplain, Spokane Fire Department

A Note From the Author

"*I am so out of control!*" And I love the way that sounds. But don't misunderstand—I am in no way reckless, dangerous, self-destructive, crazy, or anything even close. I am simply so out of control of my life and circumstances that I live in an absolutely peaceful and joyful way. The trials I have experienced the past seven years allow me to write this book from firsthand experience. The list you are about to read illustrates how I suffered much in a short period of time. So when I say I have been broken and depressed, crushed and bewildered, and that I know what suffering is, I speak the truth. But it also should help you understand, as you read this book, that giving God complete control of my life did not happen without a battle of my will.

Here is a list of the major heart-related medical procedures and surgeries I endured from September 2001 until this writing in 2008. It does not include the myriad of problems and issues with doctors, appointments, nurses, travel, insurance, and finances. (*You can find a Glossary of the medical phrases below on page 195*)

September 2001	Heart angioplasty, stent in main artery, clear left artery
October 2001	Brachytherapy and stent (two separate angioplasties in one day)

December 2001	Heart angioplasty, diagonal artery stent
January 2002	Heart angioplasty
February 2002	Heart angioplasty, main and left artery
February 2002	Open-heart surgery, double bypass, complications, two surgeries in one day, critical condition
July 2002	Heart angioplasty
August 2002	Traveled to NYC, heart angioplasty, main artery ballooned, two stents placed, two angioplasties in one week
September 2002	Heart angioplasty
October 2002	Heart angioplasty, four stents are 50% under deployed, one is blocking the main artery
October 2002	Heart angioplasty, rotablation, brachytherapy, anemic, blood transfusion
November 2002	Attempted cardiac ablation, rescheduled for December
December 2002	Ablation and pacemaker
January 2003	Main artery 90% blocked, ballooned/rotablation
January 2003	Traveled to San Diego, heart angioplasty
March 2003	Heart angioplasty
April 2003	Surgery, clean out scar tissue, re-cut sternum bone and put back together
June 2003	Heart angioplasty to find 98% blockage in middle of main artery
June 2003	Heart angioplasty to clear out blockage and another stent placed

July 2004	ER visit—severe tachycardia
August 2003	Heart angioplasty
October 2003	Heart angioplasty
December 2003	Surgery in PA—mini thoracotomy to inject FGF-1 Growth Hormone, experimental surgery
February 2004	Heart angioplasty, main artery 99% blocked
February 2004	Heart angioplasty, rotablation and brachytherapy
March 2004	Heart angioplasty
May 2004	Heart angioplasty, partial occlusion of artery–no intervention
August 2004	Heart angioplasty, artery 100% occluded–no intervention
September 2004	Heart angioplasty, two blockages in main artery–two more stents
September 2004	Heart angioplasty, two blockages in main artery–two more stents
October 2004	Heart angioplasty
December 2004	Heart angioplasty
April 2005	ER, went into cardiac arrest two times, almost died (read about my experience with death in chapter 1)
April 2005	Heart angioplasty, pre-heart transplant
July 2005	Heart transplant!
January 2006	Cytomegalovirus (CMV) detected, only treatment is chemotherapy
February 2006	CMV returns, back on chemotherapy
May 2006	CMV returns, go on a stronger chemotherapy, in hospital four weeks

October 2006	CMV returns, in hospital four weeks, then on chemotherapy at home for three months
November 2007	Broken right leg and knee

If you made it through this list, you can begin to understand why I titled this book *A Heart Like Mine*. But keep in mind, I am here to encourage those of you who read it to see that God gives us all a portion of faith—enough to make it through the toughest of trials and to emerge triumphant.

Cindy

Here are three anchor verses God gave me early on in my illness. Use these to steady yourself as you find God's will for your life:

Deal courageously, and the LORD
shall be with the good.

2 Chronicles 19:11b KJV

¤ ¤ ¤

Do not grieve, for the joy of the
LORD is your strength.

Nehemiah 8:10b NIV

¤ ¤ ¤

Beware of turning to evil, which you
seem to prefer to affliction.

Job 36:21 NIV

Introduction

In August of 2001, my husband John, my son Jonathan, and I went on an all-day canoe trip with a group of people from our church paddling the Coeur d'Alene River near Cataldo, Idaho. The day was perfect—we laughed, swam, explored, and raced to the end of our trek, each fighting to take first place. I loved the wilderness and challenge of almost constant rowing on a river that had already began its descent into fall and winter.

A few weeks later, pulling pressure and pain in my chest sent me to my family doctor. I thought I had injured some muscles while canoeing. But after three appointments and two emergency room visits, I was admitted into the advanced cardiac care unit of our local hospital. As I sat on the edge of the hospital bed, I thought, *This is a mistake. Why would they admit me for heart problems? I'm sure I just pulled some muscles*. I stared pensively at the flyers on the bulletin board describing discharge instructions after open-heart surgery.

I never considered the possibility of something being wrong with my heart. I was healthy, had low cholesterol, never smoked or drank, had no family history of heart disease, no high blood pressure, and was a healthy weight. I was content with life and filled my days with raising my son, loving my husband, volunteering for ministry, enjoying church outings, gardening, and loving all that I did.

On September 18, 2001, however, a surreal event changed everything. I nearly missed having a massive heart attack and began my induction into the world of heart disease. The first of numerous heart angioplasties left me with a stent in my main artery. After this first encounter I thought, *Okay, I can handle this, it's over now*. But it was only the beginning of a process that has changed my life forever. A rare genetic anomaly took away the vibrant health I once enjoyed. This process is unremitting, and I could choose to lapse into despair. Instead, I opted to lean into the challenge and take this as an opportunity to become stronger. And my life has been forever changed.

What if today you were presented with a unique opportunity that would change your life forever? An opportunity that would allow you to become a stronger person emotionally and spiritually, and cause you to rapidly develop the ability to conquer all the failures, temptations, trials, and painful aspects of your life. Not only would you emerge the victor over all the tragedy around you, but in the process, people who know you and people you encounter will also be empowered with your new strength.

This new change in you would be so powerful that you would never want to go back to your old life. Once overwhelmed by daily struggles with finances, relationships, jobs, marriage, children, health, etc., you now realize how easily these troubles can be eliminated. Each morning you awake to a new day of promise and actually look forward to living your life fully and wholly without the weight of dread hanging over you. Would you welcome this opportunity? Would you be willing to accept an offer like this?

Who would turn down such a freeing power? Given the many weights that burden each of us on a daily basis, no one would walk away from this chance without at the very least finding out what was involved. For most people, a change like this cannot just evolve. Although some people appear to be triumphant and godly, spiritual giants without failure, there will always be something in life that can dismantle their stature.

This process is custom tailored for each human being God has created. Unique and special to Him, every person on earth has a plan created for the good of their soul and the strengthening of their purpose here on earth. No process that would bring such power and victory in our lives can ever be accomplished without painfully removing the hindrances birthed in each of our souls. Human nature and finite minds are not able to see or comprehend the well-chosen plan God has mapped out for us. And once we find out the cost—many, if not all, would turn down the offer.

I knew nothing of this unfolding before it began in me. I thought my life was going along just fine. I figured I had grown close enough to God to the point that I understood what was expected of me and could handle whatever came my way. I was secure in my spiritual state and confident I could surrender to anything asked of me. I even accepted my failures as training and envisioned myself getting up after a defeat, shaking off the dust, and continuing on my merry way.

When trials came my way, I staggered a bit, even falling from the pressure. But clutching the Word of God and using prayer to fortify my soul, I believed I could recover from each setback completely. I looked upon people falling apart from tragedy in their lives and ran to their rescue whenever I could—eager to share my strength. Little did I know I had not even begun to tap into the power God had reserved for me. The process begins at birth and does not end until we are complete: "Being confident of this, that he who began a good work in you will carry it on to completion until the day of Christ Jesus" (Philippians 1:6 NASB). The day of Christ Jesus has not come and when we "see" Him, then we will know the work is complete. For now, the process continues in each of us, like seasons of refining. When we are ready, yet unknowingly to us, God changes the direction we are going and a season of intense training takes over. This design can bring us to what we desire to have in our lives, but would never willingly enter into.

My opportunity to reach higher ground emerged from the heart disease that has almost killed me more than once. I would never have chosen this path. My offer presented a scenario I would have easily walked away from given a choice. Who would accept the wealth of such an opportunity if it meant living with the threat of fatality from heart disease at an early age of 40?

> "For many of us, spiritual growth sometimes means going down a path we would much rather detour around."[1]

There really is no ending until we meet a new beginning.

1

Chapter 1
In The Beginning

A Heart Like Mine

Of all the hearts in the world, I've only one to give.
So insecure, a desperate pulse,
racing to your embrace.
That You could want me and seek me,
is more than words could ever say.
That You would love me and see in me,
a pearl of price thrown away.

A heart like mine, how could it be worthy,
that You'd find,
A way to redeem this hardened clay,
twisted and broken.
O Father God above, the wonder that You love,
A heart like mine.

Your holy hands hold me still, shaping my heart anew.
Once vacant shell now reclaimed,
offers its praise to You.
The one who searched 'til You found me,
a wounded lamb who's gone astray.

You stopped the world to recover me,
O Lamb of God, the price You'd pay for . . .

I make my promise to do the one thing I can do.
With abandon I can give, every heartbeat to You.

I was home alone one sunny, spring day in April 2005, and after not being able to eat breakfast, I tried to get down some lunch. Something was very wrong. I was off balance and felt like I was going to pass out. At first, I wasn't alarmed because many days were like that; many dreary days of battling the debilitating heart disease that kept me a prisoner in my house. I was sedated day and night to keep even the slightest activity from instigating a fatal heart attack.

But the symptoms got worse and I became so weak and dizzy I collapsed onto the couch. My heart was racing and anytime I moved I felt worse. At one point, I tried to get up, but I could no longer stand or sit up straight. It was time to get help.

I crawled to the telephone and tried to call someone to give me a ride to the ER. My routine was to call one of three girlfriends, and the first one I could reach would pick me up for the grueling ER experience. My husband John worked near the hospital. Once I was admitted, he would come over.

Often, going to the ER for another possible heart attack was almost a mundane event. One Fourth of July, some friends from California were visiting and we were all out in the front of our house, watching our neighbors' fireworks. Our kids were having fun with sparklers. But all day I struggled with chest pain and a rapid heart rate and that evening, I knew I needed to go to the ER.

"John," I called as I went into the house to change my shirt, "you need to take me to the ER. I think I may be having a heart attack." He grabbed a to-go cup for his coffee, filled it up, and we told our friends to enjoy the fireworks. "We'll be back later in the evening," I calmly stated, "if I don't get admitted."

My friend Jody was amazed, "How could you be so calm? You could be dying from a heart attack! What's wrong with you two?" She was really amazed at our indifference.

"Oh, it happens a lot. We're used to this," I reassured her. John and I didn't get back from the ER until 3:00 a.m. Jody and our son Jonathan were still up waiting for us. "I'm okay," I told them. "Just another near miss."

But on this one day in April, God put together the storyline so that I would live through what would be a very real experience with *death*.

For some reason, I couldn't reach any of my three friends and, to make matters worse, my husband John was on a plane to St. Louis, Missouri, where he had to work for a week. By now, I was starting to lose my vision and I knew I would have to call for an ambulance. I pulled myself up one more time to reach the phone and called 911.

"911, what is your emergency?" the operator asked.

"I think I'm having a heart attack," was my weak reply. Within a moment, she verified my address and told me the paramedics were on the way.

Dazed and disoriented, I was concerned that when they arrived, they would break down the front door which was locked. I couldn't pick myself up to get down the stairs, so I *slid* down and reached up to unlock the handle. I collapsed to the floor and waited. It seemed like only seconds before the ambulance, fire truck, paramedics, and police arrived.

The paramedics sat me up on the bottom of the stairs. I vaguely remember their look when they couldn't measure my blood pressure or heart rate. Before I knew it, I was on a stretcher on the front lawn and they were trying to start an IV to get fluids in me. I gazed up at the blue sky and thought, *What is all this for? I only need a ride*. At that point I was totally unaware that I was losing my grip on my life.

Shortly after getting the IV started, they got me in the ambulance. My little dog, Jackson, ran for the ambulance, jumped into the back doors, and sat next to the stretcher. Backed against the ambulance wall, he was determined to stay by my side and not let any one of those "men" touch me. Growling at the attempts to get him out, he snarled and bit at the paramedics. "We can't get him to come out!" one of them frantically complained.

"Just tell him to chase the cat," I said, "and he will run to the backyard." Nothing would work.

Finally, one of the paramedics put on thick gloves and gently grabbed him, putting him back in the house.

The ride to the ER was horrible. I was fading in and out and heaving from the urge to vomit, although there was nothing in my stomach. The ambulance finally came to an abrupt halt at the hospital where we were met by waiting ER personnel. I was wheeled quickly into an examination room and hooked up to a myriad of machines and monitors. My blood pressure dropped lower and lower from an already dangerous 65/45. My heart rate was up to 150 beats per minute and would have pushed higher if it weren't for the pacemaker implanted in my left shoulder. Although still conscious, I felt myself slipping away. I didn't know if it was all the medicines being pushed through two IV lines or the overwhelming nausea that was paralyzing me.

Suddenly, things became a blur and the loud noises of the busy ER faded. What seemed like forever to me was actually only seconds as time came to a halt. I can still see the nurses and doctors racing to work on my lifeless body. "She's coding!" one nurse yelled. "She's not breathing and we don't have a pulse!" Her panicked look is even now vivid in my mind. Yet, I was "still" and unable to do anything. It was as if I was outside of my body, watching and wondering about the outcome. One thing was sure to me—I knew I was dying.

Then what I thought was happening actually did happen. I was "hovering" above the entire scene, watching from above. Needles filled with medications and paraphernalia with wires and monitors were being hooked up to my lifeless body, all attempting to search for a sign of life. To this day, I can recollect everything that was said and done and I can still see the faces of all those desperately trying to save me.

People have asked me if I was peaceful or saw a white light. I wasn't peaceful; I was "still." But somehow I knew I was not supposed to die. I could feel God's presence and sensed a glow of light behind me. In my mind and my state of muted awareness, I said to God, "Lord, please don't let me die here in this ER all alone. Please, Lord, save me." He reassured me it wasn't time for me to go and instantly I took a much-needed breath.

I regained consciousness, yet my eyes seemed to never have closed. My arms were behind my head, a result of suffering cardiac seizures. "We thought we were going to lose you, young lady," the nurse chimed at me. Everyone was relieved, including me. I was alive.

My first thought as I transitioned from talking to God to regaining my senses was, *Oh, Lord, I have failed you. I always talk about surrendering all I am to You and yet here I was unwilling to let go and die*. But the Lord spoke to my ailing heart and He reassured me again that it was not my time to die.

¤ ¤ ¤

I listened to Bryan Duncan's song, *A Heart Like Mine*, often during my years of illness and cried both for my physical heart and my spiritual heart. I wanted my physical heart healed so I could live comfortably and independently in this world. I wanted my spiritual heart rejuvenated with strength to make my presence here on earth one of joy and peace—enabling me to rise above the pain.

"*A desperate pulse, racing to your embrace . . .*" Every beat we feel in our chest keeps us alive, but somewhere in the deepest part of our soul is another heartbeat that depends on God's redeeming touch. He can get to this spiritual heart only if we let Him. Wanting to be free of the tangled and painful circumstances we all suffer through is not enough to yield our hearts to God. We must each determine to give up the fight and let Him intervene for us. "The LORD will fight for you; you need only to be still" (Exodus 14:14 NIV).

I know how hard it is to give it up. I have always been a fighter but, like Jacob, I always seem to walk away with a limp each time I wrestle with God's will. The son of Isaac and Rebekah, Jacob was a shepherd in Canaan. His story is recounted in Genesis, chapters 25–50. In Genesis 32:25, we read how he wrestled with God all night. He was persistent, even to the point of God "touching the socket of his hip so it was wrenched" (NIV).

This story of Jacob in Genesis was a pivotal transformation in Jacob's life and his relationship with God. He realized God's love for him, knowing he should not have lived after seeing God's face. After this wrestling match, God changed Jacob's name to "Israel" meaning "he will rule as God" in the Hebrew language. This symbolic name of Jacob also attests of the path to his future generations.

Each time we wrestle with God, He wins, but we grow closer to His plan and purpose for us. He lovingly adds to our spiritual resources so our future will find us with hearts able to withstand the pressures of this world. When we are so completely evolved into His care, our own lives become redeemable for any purpose.

"I make my promise to do the one thing I can do. With abandon I can give, every heartbeat to You." With abandon we can give every heartbeat to God, and with faith we can walk securely in His strength. The Old Testament patriarch Abraham was promised much from God, but the trials he endured clouded his days. Still, he chose to remain faithful; "He staggered not at the promise of God through unbelief, but was strong in faith giving glory to God" (Romans 4:20 KJV).

Oswald Chambers, in his daily devotional *My Utmost For His Highest,* writes:

> Suppose that you have a deep "well" of hurt and trouble inside your heart, and Jesus comes and says to you, "Let not your heart be troubled . . ." (John 14:1). Would your response be to shrug your shoulders and say, "But, Lord, the well is too deep, and even You can't draw up quietness and comfort from it". . . When we get into difficult circumstances, we impoverish His ministry by saying, "Of course, He can't do anything about this." We struggle to reach the bottom of our own well, trying to get water for ourselves. Beware of sitting back, and saying, "It can't be done."[3]

When we place our lives in God's encompassing care, our resolve must include a complete trust in His provision. One day, Nancy Missler—a close friend of mine who has made a tremendous impact on my life during the past years of pain and sickness—demonstrated this trust. She sat with a friend and me one day before this friend received a heart transplant. Here was Melinda, struggling to live long enough to watch her small daughter grow up. And here I was, not knowing at what moment a heart attack could end my life.

"I wish I could give my heart to either one of you," Nancy shared with tender mercy. "I've lived my life already. I don't need it." Her genuine offer to sacrifice her own life for us is evidence of the work God had done in her long before. Nancy relinquished control of her life and allowed God to build her up so she could build up those around her. Her obvious freedom to offer her heart to us was affirmation of her trust in God.

After my near-death experience that day, and my encounter with God, I realized that a fear I had held onto for years—even as a Christian—was now gone. Although I knew about all the promises of God and what the Bible said about being a Christian and facing death, I was still afraid to die. But those few moments gave me an unexplainable peace. I no longer fear what may happen, how I may die, or what I might suffer. As a child of God, I am secure in His safety.

And during the week I spent in the hospital after my incident in the ER, I enjoyed seeing the reaction of visitors as they entered my room. A coworker from my husband's office expressed his surprise that I was sitting up in bed smiling and joking around the very next day. Even my doctor said, "You are really in good spirits for someone who just went through what you did." The question each of their reactions revealed was, "Where does your help come from?"

As I lay in the hospital bed one night unable to stop my mind from scattered thoughts, I prayed and asked the Lord to show me precisely how to explain this "help" He had given me. The explanation God presented to me was a simple concept.

Do you remember preparing for a test in grade school or college? You may recall the uneasy feeling when the paper is placed in your hand and the questions stare at you like empty expectations. Not knowing the material leaves you unable to answer quickly and decisively. On the other hand, preparing for the test and knowing the subject from all aspects allows you to breeze through each question with ease and confidence. Like practicing a sport, rehearsing a musical piece, or reciting a speech over and over, being intimate with your subject provides you with the skill needed to succeed.

What does wise King Solomon from the Old Testament in the Bible say about this illustration? "If the ax is dull and its edge unsharpened, more strength is needed, but skill will bring success" (Ecclesiastes 10:10 NIV). Webster's Dictionary defines "skill" as "a learned power of doing something competently." Our learned power, our skill, is to know God so deeply and so confidently, that in intense times of trouble we easily draw near to Him and allow Him to carry out His predetermined plan. That complete surrender frees us up to succeed, to pass the test before us with little effort.

Where does *your* help come from? Consistently reading the Word of God, fervently praying, and knowing Him so well that your *skill* is found in Him. Feed your mind and your soul with things of heaven, renewing yourself from the hurting world around you.

I had to do this. I found myself so close to death so many times that if I couldn't perceive my strength in God, I would not have lived through all that I did. And after nearly four years of close calls, the day came when I had nothing else to rely on except God.

On Wednesday, July 13, 2005, my heart surgeon came in to see me and essentially told me we were out of options. "We won't be able to get you a donor heart for at least a year," he told me, "and you don't have a year." His outlook was not good and the only viable answer was to consider leaving me in the hospital on IV medications for as long as it took to get a donor heart—months that could turn into a year or more! Although Ventricular Assist Devices (VAD) can be used as a "bridge" to a heart transplant, he told me the surgery would be too dangerous and he did not want to pursue the option unless there was no other choice.

I woke up at 6:30 the next morning, Thursday, July 14. When I went to the sink to brush my teeth, I saw a note for the nurses "NPO" meaning "nothing by mouth." The thought came to me, *He got a heart for me; I just know he did.* The nurses were coming in and out for various reasons but couldn't tell me anything. Knowing me so well and following my plight for the past three and a half years, they were bursting at the seams to tell me what was happening. But they didn't have to—I knew.

At 8:30, the heart surgeon came in. "Sign on the dotted line," he said as he placed a consent form in front of me. I saw the words *Heart Transplant* written in on the permission line, but I still had to ask.

"What for?" I wanted to hear it from him.

"You want a new heart, don't you?" He explained to me that a 28-year-old woman had died who was an organ donor, but the transplant centers in our Northwest region had all turned down her heart for donation. Her heart needed two valves repaired and it also had a hole in its inner wall called the septum. Once a donor heart is rejected, my surgeon is the only doctor in the Northwest who is willing to take a rejected heart and actually repair it, making it workable for a transplant in someone like me, desperately needing help.

After he explained to me the repairs it needed, I asked, "What makes you think this heart will work for me if all the other transplant centers turned it down?"

"Because this is the one the Lord has for you," he replied with confidence.

"I totally trust you." My reply was also confident, as I knew God had ordained this miracle.

He left the room and a barrage of nurses and technicians began the preparations for surgery. With a surge of emotion, John and I watched out the window of my hospital room as the MedStar helicopter left with the doctor, his own equipment, and his team of operating personnel for a small airport five minutes away. From there they would board a Lear jet that would swiftly fly them to the University Hospital in Seattle where my surgeon would inspect and possibly repair the donor heart.

Once I was in the waiting room of the OR, my transplant coordinator explained to me that they would be putting me under anesthesia, but I could actually wake up back in my room, the whole thing a false alarm. "If the doctor decides the heart cannot be repaired, you may wake up to find out nothing was done." She wanted me to be prepared, yet inside I knew this was it. This was what God had planned and prayer was being answered.

As the IVs were started, I looked at John and my last words to him were, "When I wake up and see you, I will say 'I made it!'" Then everything went dark. In what seemed like a few seconds—but actually almost ten hours later—I woke up in intensive care only long enough to fulfill my promise. "I made it!" I said before my eyes closed back into a deep sleep. How grateful I was to know it was over and I was alive! My surgeon had repaired the heart, flown back to Spokane, and at 5:30 p.m. placed it in my chest from which my own heart had been removed. He explained to me later that it was the most repairs he had ever done to a transplanted heart. The operating report even stated that without all the techniques needed to get a transplanted heart to start pumping, this heart began beating as soon as it was placed in my chest and my own blood began to flow through it. It was as if it was meant to be part of me.

The medical center where my transplant was performed, Sacred Heart Medical Center, in Spokane, Washington, boasts the highest success rates for patients surviving a heart transplant at the one year tally and the three year tally. According to an article published by The Living Legacy Foundation in Seattle, Washington,

> The program that began in 1989 [and] now posts survival rates that routinely exceed national levels," said Dr. Timothy Icenogle, the 54-year-old cardiac surgeon who directs the program.

> *Only* one of 32 patients died after receiving heart transplants at Sacred Heart between January 2003 and June 2005, according to data released last month from a national transplant registry.
>
> That's a success rate of nearly 97 percent after one year, compared with nearly 88 percent nationwide, and more than 95 percent after three years, compared with less than 80 percent nationally, according to the Scientific Registry of Transplant Recipients (SRTR).[4]

Not only was I in a place where the survival rates are the highest, but my surgeon is a man who looks to the Lord for his ability to save lives:

> "I don't believe in the providence of luck," Icenogle said. "I believe in mathematical probability and the providence of the Lord."[5]

I still wake up each day with awe that I am alive. The strange part is knowing that someone else's heart is beating in my chest. It's almost unreal—yet I considered, at times, how a family or husband somewhere was willing to donate this young women's heart to save the life of another. (Read about my heart donor and her family in chapter 7.)

Jesus laid down His life for us so we could have eternal life. No one person on earth can do this for any of us. But as God's children, we can lay down our own lives for others out of love:

> This is the message you heard from the beginning: We should love one another. We know that we have passed from death to life, because we love our brothers. Anyone who does not love remains in death. This is how we know what love is: Jesus Christ laid down his

> life for us. And we ought to lay down our lives for our brothers. If anyone has material possessions and sees his brother in need but has no pity on him, how can the love of God be in him? (1 John 11,14,16-17 NIV).

When I think back to the very beginning, I never comprehended what was ahead of me. Over a period of five years, I was an inpatient 54 times at the hospital where I had my heart transplant! I was always admitted on the cardiac unit and, sadly, occupied the same rooms more than once.

Many times, I glanced up at the pale green walls and gazed angrily at the flyers posted on the bulletin board. Their colored pages stared defiantly at me: "Open Heart Surgery Class," "Heart Healthy Nutrition Class," "Home Care for Bypass Patients," "Cardiac Rehabilitation." I was prisoner to their defiance, prisoner to the myriad of bottles dripping fluids into my veins, prisoner to the fear that consumed me.

The very first procedure happened so fast, I hardly remember being scared or even sure of what was about to happen to me. But on that day, as I waited in my room for the transport people to take me to surgery, I looked at my husband John and spoke words I never expected to utter. "I have one last request," I stated through quivering lips. John turned away, unable to look into my fearful eyes. "You have to promise me you will not be angry with God if He takes me today."

There was no reaction from him. No answer. He couldn't even look at me. Still I insisted and he turned to look at me, his face revealing his pain. I had my answer. He would forever hold my words in his mind, but at that moment it wasn't possible for him to guarantee such a promise. I was okay with that and settled my head back into the pillows.

Finally, I was wheeled to the heart catheterization lab where I was prepped for the procedure. I was semi-awake, but conscious enough to realize what was happening. The two doctors working on me found the blockage more severe than they thought and the seriousness of it prompted them to prepare me for open-heart surgery. At the last minute, another cardiologist was called in who, after several painstaking attempts, was able to clear the blockage and insert a stent (a woven metallic tube) to enlarge the artery. When they were done, I think the surgeons and assistants—five in all—wanted to clap with relief and surprise.

Afterwards, the cardiologist informed me that if I had suffered a heart attack, I would not have survived. The blockages were in the worst place and they were extensive. In fact, these particular blockages are called "widow makers" because they are more common in men and usually lead to death.

Later, back in my room, I tried to understand what had just happened to me. This was all new. I never had to worry about heart disease before. For me, those blocked arteries loomed in the hazy balance of keeping the blood flow sufficient to supply my heart muscle with much needed blood and oxygen. I knew that at any time something could go wrong and, within minutes, I could be gone.

The ensuing months, and then years, after this first incident earned me a title in the heart catheterization lab: "The Legend." No one could believe how many times I was wheeled into the procedure room to clear out yet another blockage. Within the first three years after developing heart disease, I went through more than 30 catheterizations.

Unfortunately, I became popular on 6-South, the Advanced Cardiac Care Unit. It was my second home. The staff, whether nurses or janitorial staff, all knew me well. And sometimes they became so connected with me, it made it hard for them to watch me fade away as my heart was pummeled with one blockage after another.

During one hospital visit, my blood pressure began to drop as my heart rate quickened to a dangerous level. The heart monitor alarms went off and, within seconds, every nurse available charged into the room. My bed was tilted back and medicines were pushed through my IVs.

One nurse I had become closely attached to left the room, face pale with fear. Later that afternoon, she came back in to apologize.

"I am so sorry I ran out," she explained. "I couldn't take it. I didn't want to lose you and I was afraid you might die right there." The nurses are trained to separate themselves from these times, and they are normally not allowed to leave the room when a patient is in danger of "coding," a term used when someone is close to dying.

"I understand," I assured her. Her love and concern made me realize how connected the staff had become. It also was part of a realization that a person's heart is more than muscle and blood vessels. My physical heart was breaking, but it began an awareness in me that the heart is more than just a pump, and it can also be broken emotionally and spiritually.

Can a heart really be broken? It's often considered that a person's heart is the place where the most cherished memories are held. We talk freely about our heart aching for someone far away, or our hearts going out to others when they are hurting. How do our hearts go out? Do we control them with our minds, or is our heart the central control system? The heart is considered merely a pump by the medical profession, a mass of muscle, vessels, and networked electrical pathways, pulsing blood through our bodies. But think about this—of all the parts in our physical bodies, there is only one heart and we cannot live without it. Many, if not most, of our other body parts and systems can be damaged, destroyed, or shut down and we can still live. Many people are missing multiple physical abilities, yet they live productive and fulfilling lives.

Many writers and literary works refer often to the heart, giving it a grand place of distinction. Not merely the physical heart, but the heart as its own entity; its own, independent system of emotions, memories, and controls.

Also prevalent in literature, prose, and music, is the concept of a broken heart as penned in an old hymn written in the early 1900s by Thomas Dennis, an assistant pastor in Haslemere, Surrey, England:

Have you read that He saved the dying thief,
When hanging on the tree,
Who looked with pleading eyes and said,
"Dear Lord, remember me?"
Have you read that He looked to heaven and said,
'Tis finished—'twas for thee?
Have you ever said, I thank you Lord,
For giving Thy life for me?

He died of a broken heart for you,
He died of a broken heart;
Oh, wondrous love! For you, for me—
He died of a broken heart.

"The Broken Heart" by Thomas Dennis

Could Jesus have a broken heart? His Father did. Genesis 6:6 tells us, "The LORD was sorry that He had made man on the earth, and He was grieved in His heart" (NASB). Dennis's description of the broken heart of Jesus echoes the important place one's heart takes in our lives as so often mentioned in the Holy Scriptures.

In her book, *The Heart Speaks*, renowned cardiologist Dr. Mimi Guarneri describes the newly discovered place the heart takes in the body's systems of communication:

> In ancient Greece, Aristotle believed that since the heart was "central, mobile, and hot, and well supplied with structures which served to communicate between it and the rest of the body," it was most suitable to be the seat of the soul.
>
> No matter which view is taken, the heart possesses special attributes that give it supremacy over the brain as the key organ for our survival. It is formed first and stops last. By the sixth week of pregnancy, when the fetus is no bigger than a marble, the cardiac muscle has already formed and begun its initial fluttering movements. Life can continue without the brain, but not once the heart has stopped.
>
> The heart is also exquisitely sensitive to emotions. An angry or fearful thought changes the heart rate variability (HRV) patter—the beat-to-beat variability between each heartbeat—which sets the pace for the brain and respiratory system.
>
> It's long been known that emotions have a physiological impact on our bodies. ...But what if it's not the brain telling the heart what to feel, but the heart informing the rest of the body? What if changing the mind actually involves changing the heart?[6]

With such a strong association of the heart's upper role now prevalent in the medical community, it's no wonder physicians haven't realized its potential as the Word of God does. Many scriptures refer to the different aspects of the heart. You cannot read about the heart God describes as being the center of our souls without reading about how it also leads and controls our minds, decisions, and lives. It is the most talked about subject in the Bible.

Do not let kindness and truth leave you; bind them around your neck, write them on the tablet of your heart (Proverbs 3:3 NASB).

The heart can have integrity: Then God said to him in the dream, "Yes, I know that in the integrity of your heart you have done this, and I also kept you from sinning against Me; therefore I did not let you touch her (Genesis 20:6 NASB).

The heart can be glad: Aaron the Levite? I know that he speaks fluently. And moreover, behold, he is coming out to meet you; when he sees you, he will be glad in his heart (Genesis 4:14b NASB).

The heart can be evil and sinful: For from within, out of the heart of men, proceed the evil thoughts, fornications, thefts, murders, adulteries, deeds of coveting and wickedness, as well as deceit, sensuality, envy, slander, pride and foolishness. All these evil things proceed from within and defile the man (Mark 7: 21-23, NASB).

The heart contains life: Watch over your heart with all diligence, for from it flow the springs of life (Proverbs 4:23 NASB).

The heart can be hard: His heart is as hard as a stone, even as hard as a lower millstone (Job 41:24 NASB).

> *The heart can be renewed*: Moreover, I will give you a new heart and put a new spirit within you; and I will remove the heart of stone from your flesh and give you a heart of flesh (Ezekiel 36:26 NASB).
>
> For God, who said, "Light shall shine out of darkness," is the One who has shone in our hearts to give the Light of the knowledge of the glory of God in the face of Christ (2 Corinthians 4:6 NASB).

Hundreds of scriptures describe the heart as much more than simply a physical part of our body. As Dr. Guarneri illustrates, "Forgiveness, optimism, gratitude, [love]—these topics would have been dismissed as irrelevant when I was in medical school. Now they are increasingly subjects for serious scientific investigation, as much a part of the heart disease equation as blood cholesterol levels."

During one of my dreary hospital incarcerations, instigated by a near fatal heart attack, a dear friend came to visit me. She chatted for a bit and then handed me a book she read recently and thought I might like to read.

The title startled me: *Waking the Dead* by John Eldredge. *Waking the Dead?* What kind of a book was that for someone like me, in the hospital holding on for life? But this book dissipated the dreariness of those lonely days.

John Eldredge, like Dr. Guarneri, speaks of the central role our heart plays physically and spiritually.

> The heart is central. That we would even need to be reminded of this only shows how far we have fallen from the life we were meant to live—or how powerful the spell has been. The subject of the heart is addressed in the Bible more than any other topic—more than

> works or service, more than belief or obedience, more than money, and even more than worship. Maybe God knows something we've forgotten.
>
> The Bible sees the heart as the source of all creativity, courage, and conviction. It is the source of our faith, our hope, and of course, our love. It is the "wellspring of life" within (Prov. 4:23), the very essence of our existence, the center of our being, the fount of our life.
>
> There is no escaping the centrality of the heart. God knows that; it's why he made it the central theme of the Bible, just as he placed the physical heart in the center of the human body. The heart is central; to find our lives, we must make it central again.[7]

As important as the heart is to our physical lives, it can also be broken—physically and spiritually. In Isaiah 27:11, God shows us a picture of how easily this can be done: "When its twigs are dry, they are broken off and women come and make fires with them. For this is a people without understanding; so their Maker has no compassion on them, and their Creator shows them no favor." The Hebrew word here for a bush with fragile, easily broken twigs is *leb shabar*—*leb* representing "heart" and *shabar* meaning broken.

Two of my favorite verses about God's love to the brokenhearted are found in Psalms and Isaiah:

> The LORD is close to the brokenhearted, and saves those who are crushed in spirit (Psalm 34:18 NIV).

> The Spirit of the LORD GOD is upon me; because the LORD hath anointed me to preach good tidings unto the meek; he hath sent me to bind up the brokenhearted,

to proclaim liberty to the captives, and the opening of the prison to them that are bound (Isaiah 61:1 KJV).

Can a heart actually be broken physically?

Taking into consideration the wisdom of the poets and philosophers, doctors are now reporting that the sudden death of someone you love can cause a broken heart. In fact, the condition "broken heart syndrome" is now being officially recognized by doctors the world over as reported by cardiologist Dr. Ilan Wittstein, M.D of The Johns Hopkins University School of Medicine:

> Shocking news, such as learning of the unexpected death of a loved one, has been known to cause catastrophic events, such as a heart attack.
>
> Now, researchers at Johns Hopkins have discovered that sudden emotional stress can also result in severe but reversible heart muscle weakness that mimics a classic heart attack. Patients with this condition, called stress cardiomyopathy but known colloquially as "broken heart" syndrome, are often misdiagnosed with a massive heart attack when, indeed, they have suffered from a days-long surge in adrenalin (epinephrine) and other stress hormones that temporarily "stun" the heart.
>
> After observing several cases of "broken heart" syndrome at Hopkins hospitals - most of them in middle-aged or elderly women - we realized that these patients had clinical features quite different from typical cases of heart attack, and that something very different was happening," says Wittstein. "These cases were, initially, difficult to explain because most of the patients

were previously healthy and had few risk factors for heart disease.

While the folklore of "broken heart" syndrome has been around for decades, the prevalence of the condition remains unknown. According to Wittstein, some reports exist, mainly from Japan, and describe similar syndromes, but no biochemical analyses have previously been performed that link the condition to elevated catecholamine levels. The researchers contend that while stress cardiomyopathy is not as common as a typical heart attack, it likely occurs more frequently than doctors realize. They expect its numbers to increase as more physicians learn to recognize the syndrome's unique clinical features.[8]

> Who has put wisdom in the mind? Or who has given understanding to the heart? (Job 38:36, NKJV)

Understanding the heart physically, emotionally, and spiritually is the beginning of understanding what makes each one of us who we are. And once we find the origin of our own heartaches, we can begin to grasp what we need to overcome the individual trials breaking our hearts.

Chapter 2
Chasing the Wind

February 2002, five months after my first heart attack, and six heart catheterizations and two stents later, I again found myself quickly going downhill. My worst fear was no longer having another heart attack but what the doctors would think when I told them I was worse again. The last instructions I received were, "Don't call us unless you have symptoms similar to the first incident in September." The absurdity of so many cardiac issues was baffling to most of the medical staff caring for me.

Okay, I thought, *I'll wait until it gets bad. I won't call them unless I know something is really wrong.*

Then at 2:00 a.m. on February 16, 2002, the chest pain was so bad it woke me from a deep sleep. I jolted up and the pain pierced my chest, making its way up into my neck and jaw. As I stumbled out of bed, I almost collapsed from the shock. I made it to the kitchen and grasped the bottle of nitroglycerin pills, quickly placing one under my tongue. As the nitro melted into my bloodstream, a rush of relief cascaded down my chest. The pain lessened and I could breathe without gasping. But the results lasted only15 minutes and by the time I took the third pill, I knew it was time to call the doctor.

I woke John up and told him what had happened, then I called the emergency number for my cardiologist's office. When the answering service put me through, I spoke with a doctor I didn't know. But he certainly knew who I was. After explaining what was happening, his reply brought panic to my already frazzled nerves. "You can go to the ER but I don't think it's your heart," he said smugly.

"What do you mean you don't think it's my heart?" I was obviously provoked. He refused to give me a reason. I dug my heels in and insisted I would not go unless he told me why he didn't think it was my heart. "Why should I go if it isn't my heart?" I retorted. "Why waste everyone's time and money. Besides, I hate going to the ER." We argued back and forth until he finally got frustrated enough to give me an answer.

"I don't want to argue this all night. All right, I'll tell you why I don't think it's your heart. With your history of having symptoms for no reason, I think this is just psychological. But you can go to the ER anyway."

His reasoning made me so angry I cried and handed the telephone to John. After a few minutes he hung up and took me to the ER. But instead of making the 20-minute drive to the ER where the Heart Institute was, I had him take me to our local hospital.

At the ER I was poked, prodded, and x-rayed. A dose of morphine and some nitroglycerin were pushed through the IV, yet I was still having severe symptoms. All the tests came back normal—but that always seemed to happen. Still, the ER doctor wanted me transported to the ER at the hospital downtown. She telephoned the cardiologist who was on call and told him she would prefer that I was transported by ambulance to the Sacred Heart Medical Center ER. His reply shocked her. "Oh, just cap off the IV and have her husband drive her. I'm sure she's fine. In fact, send her to admitting instead of the ER. I'll check in on her after she gets to a room." Even though this made the ER doctor very uneasy, John and I left and drove to the other hospital.

We got there at 5:00 a.m. Our instructions were to go straight to admitting but no one was at the desk. John grabbed a wheelchair and pushed me down the empty hallways to try to find an admitting clerk. I sat in the wheelchair watching the dimly lit pictures on the colorless walls sail by as John desperately searched for anyone who could tell us where to go. I grabbed my chest, as the pain came and went in waves, warning me that something was wrong.

Finally, a security guard stopped us and asked us where we were going. “I’m really not sure,” John replied, bewildered. “We’re supposed to find someone to admit my wife. She’s having chest pain.” The guard escorted us to the ER where I was checked in and then waited for someone to transport me to a room. Already familiar with the Advanced Cardiac Care Unit, I wondered what nurses were working that morning.

Once up in the room, all the check-in procedures began: Medical history? What medicines are you taking? Who is your doctor? etc., etc. I answered the questions as tears welled up in my eyes. I was tired and worn-out. *Why won’t they believe me?* I wondered.

After all the paperwork and blood work were done, I was hooked up to the standard heart monitor that relayed my information remotely to the nurse’s station. My heartbeat, EKG, and heart rhythm would be displayed on a TV-like monitor along with those of almost 50 other patients. A nurse sat in front of the pulsating monitors for an entire shift, watching for any abnormalities.

At 7:00 a.m. I sat on the uncomfortable hospital bed feeling as inanimate as the room around me. The doctor on call during the night came into the room and sat next to me. John listened as he spoke to me in a monotone voice. “I know you think I don’t believe you, but you know, psychology can cause you to have symptoms if you are always scared that something could go wrong.”

I looked at him and replied defiantly, "When you get a degree in psychology, then I will let you tell me what you think. But I don't believe a cardiologist is required to also major in psychology." After my cutting response, he told me he would be doing a heart catheterization early that afternoon and left. I cried quietly.

Several hours passed before I was prepped and wheeled into the cardiac catheterization lab. The doctor arrived and the monitors above my head displayed the inside of my chest. As he threaded the catheter through my femur artery and filled the vessels on top of my heart with dye, I watched anxiously for any indications of a blockage. I had just enough anesthesia in me to be awake and aware of what was being done.

The dye filled my arteries and then at one point, I could no longer see any evidence of the artery. I knew there was a blockage and I knew it was bad. In fact, both my main left artery and a branch coming from it were not filling with dye. I looked at the doctor and his face revealed his regret.

"I guess I should have believed you." He spoke with a heavy sigh and left the room. I never saw him again.

The only option given to me was open-heart surgery. I was infused with tubes delivering medicines that all came together into a main IV site. They kept me stable but would only suffice until something more was done.

So many times I felt like I was chasing answers down empty pathways. It was like Lewis Carroll's Alice in Wonderland when Alice first encountered the White Rabbit:

> Down, down, down. Would the fall never come to an end! "I wonder how many miles I've fallen by this time?" she said aloud. "I must be getting somewhere near the centre of the earth."[9]

From the very first cardiologist, there was a hesitancy to believe my symptoms were real. Time after time, I found myself arguing with staff and attempting to persuade doctors that my symptoms were valid. At one point I actually paid a Christian psychologist to do an assessment testing of my state of mind so I could prove to the doctors I was not "creating" my symptoms. I passed the testing with high grades and in his words I was "a high energy, social individual that shows an ability to be assertive when necessary. In my opinion, there is no evidence in my clinical interviews or in the psychological test administered to indicate that she has any psychological etiology for her physical symptoms."

Only one month after my very first procedure, the impending symptoms returned. When I contacted the cardiologist's office, I was met with a cold resistance from the staff. Several nurses spoke to me by phone and explained away my returning symptoms as normal. After I persisted, they finally ordered further testing.

After all the tests were done—including another nuclear stress test where I walked on a treadmill and the response of my heart was measured, I asked the receptionist when I would hear back about the results. I wanted to speak to the doctor, or at least the nurse. I was informed I could talk to a doctor only if I had an appointment. "After all," she told me, "we have too many patients to deal with." I was informed I would have to wait until my November 26 appointment.

"That's not for another month and a half. Do you mean I can't talk to any one of the doctors here unless I have an appointment?" I was becoming anxious and could feel my emotions welling up inside of me.

But the receptionist would not budge. Her attitude was insensitive and uncaring. I began to cry. I found myself explaining over and over that this was all new to me and I just wanted to know if the symptoms I was experiencing were to be expected. If I had not been feeling so bad or if I was told what was happening to me was normal, I would not have asked to speak to a doctor. All I wanted was a few minutes with any one. Three nurses had already given me different opinions, so I wanted some reassurance.

My mind raced with thoughts—angry thoughts. This was not simply a bad tooth or a broken bone. This was a close encounter with a possible fatal heart attack. I felt that the people in the office were so used to the "routine," they forgot that new patients are scared, confused, and upset and might need more consideration.

With all the emotions I felt that day came the realization that the medical community was made up of people, and people will fail. Many of my appointments would turn into painful disappointments as time after time I was treated with "protocol." Even though, as a Christian, I chose to be patient, enduring, and understanding, I found myself having to fight for proper health care. And, unfortunately, health care in the United States is on the decline.

> If the United States spends more on health care than any other nation, why isn't our health care system venerated as the best in the world? It is questions like these that inspire the work of Dr. Christopher J. L. Murray, director of the Institute for Health Metrics and Evaluation (IHME) at the University of Washington and professor of global health at the UW School of Medicine and School of Public Health and Community Medicine. University of Washington Television.[10]

In Dr. Murray's research of healthcare in the U.S., he came to this conclusion:

> The United States spends the most of any country on health care by far, yet we're ranked 30th to 40th in the world in terms of quality of public health.

> According to the Center for Disease Control, there is an average of 27 doctors for every 10,000 people in the United States. The average in larger cities is much higher, with New York averaging 37 doctors per 10,000 people and Washington, DC averaging as high as 74 doctors per 10,000. The dramatic difference of health care in varying geographical areas can mean the difference between quality of life for some and life or death for others.[11]

Still, patient satisfaction, as reported in the same article, is no better when there is higher doctor-to-patient per capita ratios. According to Dr. Murray, "Studies of individual hospitals have likewise shown that while the doctor-patient ratio varies widely from place to place, more doctors do not mean better care."

Why is patient satisfaction so low? Why do more doctors choose larger cities over rural areas?

> Like anyone else, doctors want to live in places where they can earn high incomes, enjoy cultural and leisure activities, and send their children to good schools. Doctors migrate to states on lists of "Best Places to Live": Forty of the top 100 cities with "strong arts, cultural programs, and higher education" were in the ten states with the highest per capita number of doctors.[12]

After six years of heart disease, 59 inpatient hospital stays, dozens of doctor appointments and procedures, two open-heart surgeries, a heart transplant, and numerous complications, I can say firsthand that part of the problem lies with a decline in compassion and genuine care. Although doctors are mandated to uphold the Hippocratic Oath, I believe the modern-day interpretation of it has dwindled from its original purpose and an integral part of it has been forgotten: "I will remember that there is art to medicine as well as science, and that warmth, sympathy, and understanding may outweigh the surgeon's knife or the chemist's drug."

The Word of God says about these days on earth: "Because of the increase of wickedness, the love of most will grow cold" (Matthew 24:12 NIV).

In Dr. Guarneri's book, the cardiologist comments on the decadent state of patient care and how it affects relationships between doctors and their patients:

> Just like the heart, the relationship between a patient and a doctor exists within a cultural context. And in our culture at the present moment, the model is too much technology and not enough time. Therapeutic relationships with empathic family physicians have often been replaced with rushed, impersonal encounters with technicians and machines.
>
> In spite of studies that have long reported that doctors who attend to what their patients tell them have improved clinical outcomes, the constant complaint in patient satisfaction surveys is "My doctor doesn't listen to me!"
>
> Patients aren't alone in finding the quality of medical treatment disturbing. "If I'm not fast, I'm fired," a doctor friend told me.
>
> A heart can't possibly be fathomed simply through catheterization readings or cholesterol levels. The deep stories carved into the hearts of patients can be told only by them.
>
> My patients had changed me. They had shown me the importance of the heart's biography. They had taught

> me that that coronary disease is physical, spiritual, and emotional.[13]

I believe Dr. Guarneri is paving the way for doctors to combat the regression from patient care being compassionate and intuitive. She also points out the benefits of physicians who looked to God for help: "A study published in the journal of *Oncology* found that medical personnel at a cancer center in New York City who described themselves as religious were less subject than other practitioners to emotional exhaustion or 'diminished empathy.'"

Years of dealing with numerous health care settings, different physicians, and health care workers has seasoned my patience with temperance. Chuck Swindoll, in his Bible Study Guide *Hope in Hurtful Times, A Study of 1 Peter*, wants our focus not to be on the unfair treatment, but on what God would have us do when we are treated wrongly:

> And the natural tendency of the human heart is to fight back against unfair and unreasonable treatment. But Peter's point is that seeking revenge for unjust suffering is a sign of self-appointed lordship over one's affairs.[14]

Swindoll's advice?

> If you're enduring suffering right now, especially unjust suffering, it can be a dizzying experience. To keep your balance in those times, when things are swirling around you, it's important to find a fixed point and focus on it.[15]

Many painful experiences I continuously endured through all the medical issues and procedures bring me back to the verses I listed in the beginning of this book, the anchors that keep me from drowning in self-pity and anger:

> Beware of turning to evil, which you seem to prefer to affliction (Job 36:21 NIV).

> Do not grieve, for the joy of the LORD is your strength (Nehemiah 8:10b NIV).

> Deal courageously, and the LORD shall be with the good (2 Chronicles 19:11b KJV).

God wants me to be courageous, He does not want me to grieve, and He does not want me to choose evil over affliction. Many of us going through difficult times right now need to have a heavenly perspective. In James 4:13-14, the Lord shows us how our lives are not something we can hold on to: "Now listen, you who say, 'Today or tomorrow we will go to this or that city, spend a year there, carry on business and make money.' Why, you do not even know what will happen tomorrow. What is your life? You are a mist that appears for a little while and then vanishes" (NIV).

The King James Version calls our lives a "vapor" which Webster's defines as "something insubstantial," and a mist as "something that dims, obscures, or blurs."

If our lives are a mist or vapor, we cannot hold on to them, we cannot mold our future, we cannot control when our lives begin or end. These three concepts—do not turn to evil, be joyful, and be courageous—have sustained me through the many letdowns in the past years, and that continue to this very day. I sought help from doctors in my home state of Washington, and in San Diego, California; Phoenix, Arizona; New York; Pennsylvania; and as far away as Canada and Italy.

When my blockages first began, stents—small coiled, metal supports to hold open coronary arteries—were the best choice over open-heart surgery. Often, however, these stents would block up due to scar tissue from the grueling procedure of clearing out the original blockages. On the horizon were "medicated" stents that were coated with a medicine to prevent "restenosis" or recurrence of blockages after corrective surgery on a coronary artery. These drug-coated stents were approved by the U.S. Food & Drug Administration in 2003, but there were many times before they were approved that I was in desperate need of their technology.

One snowy January afternoon, I was admitted to the hospital for chest pain. With all the complications I had from prior procedures, neither I nor the doctors hardly knew what to think. After being admitted to one of my frequented rooms on 6-South, my cell phone rang. The phone call was from a doctor from Scripps Clinic in San Diego, California who was part of a three-man, doctor/friend team originating in New York. Back in August 2002, I had traveled to New York City to be examined by one of his cohorts—a doctor heading up drug-coated stents for the Johnson & Johnson Company. While there I had two angioplasties performed and two stents placed in my arteries in only two days!

Joy filled my entire being when I heard his voice on the phone. Not only is it uncommon for a doctor to call, let alone a "famous" doctor! His proposition gave me hope:

"I heard about your case and am willing to place a medicated stent in your coronary artery if you are having another blockage. The only setback is there are many protocol requirements, so you will have to be here at the hospital by 10:00 a.m. tomorrow to be eligible for the medicated stent." His voice was enough to send me into a whirlwind of determination.

"I will be there," was my confident reply. I hung up the phone, quickly explained to the nurse what was happening, and told her I wanted to be discharged.

"But I just got you in the system," she stated. "If you sign yourself out, you not only take the chance of having a heart attack, you will be considered AMA by your insurance."

"What is AMA?" I asked her.

"Against Medical Advice, and the insurance company can choose to deny payment for your time here."

"Just show me where to sign," I insisted. "I have to go."

I immediately called my husband and told him I had to be in San Diego the next morning. It was almost 6:00 p.m. However, there were no more flights to San Diego out of Spokane, Washington, where I lived. The only flight we found was out of Portland, Oregon the next morning at 5:00. I looked outside. Snow had begun to fall heavily and we were in for a bad storm.

Shortly after, John picked me up at the hospital with my 15-year-old son Jonathan, and we took him to friends where he would stay for the few days we would be gone. I had packed a quick bag with the essentials I needed, along with medical records and my medications. When we dropped Jonathan off, I watched him wave goodbye, holding back my tears: *Would I be back to see him?* We drove away in the heavy snow.

The freeway was snow-packed and covered with ice. My husband drove the speed limit, 55 mph, trying to keep our van on the road. We passed numerous vehicles that had slid off the freeway. A UPS truck sat in the middle divider, leaning dangerously to one side. I watched out the window intently, wanting to help in some way.

A few times I gasped as John almost slid off the road. "Please go lie down in the back before you really do have a heart attack!" he commanded me.

I climbed to the backseat and tried to rest my head on a pillow, but apprehension got the best of me. I made my way back to the front seat and tried to remain calm.

After a couple of hours, the foreboding snow changed to a dense fog. All we could see was the silver hood of our van reflecting what little light there was. Following a tractor trailer's lights in front of us, we continued until we reached Oregon, where the hint of sunrise began to lighten the sky and cut through the fog. It was now almost 3:30 a.m., and we had to get to the airport in Portland in time for the 5:00 a.m. flight.

Finally we pulled into the parking lot. John grabbed my bags so I would not have to carry anything as we made our way to the terminal. My heart pounded in my chest and I feared a heart attack might strike before we made it to San Diego. Reaching the gate with no time to spare, we made the flight and settled in for a two-and-a-half-hour ride. I prayed, "Oh Lord, please let us make it to the hospital on time. And please help me to survive this flight without having a heart attack."

When we landed in Portland, a friend met us at the airport where we rented a car. The plan was that we would follow him to the hospital to save time on trying to find it ourselves. I sat in the back of the rental car so I could rearrange my luggage to create a small overnight bag for the stay. I phoned my friend to let her know we were safely in San Diego and to check on Jonathan.

"Angie? Hi! It's me, Cindy. We made it here safely. How is Jonathan?" I was trying to pack my bag as I held the phone against my ear. She told me Jonathan was fine and asked when we would be arriving at the hospital. But before I could answer, the car started to veer off the freeway and pull over to the shoulder.

"Get out!" John yelled frantically at me.

"What are you doing?" I asked him.

"The car caught fire! Get out!"

"Angie, the car is on fire. I have to go. Don't worry." I hung up abruptly.

We jumped out of the car, grabbing our bags. Smoke rose from the undercarriage.

Standing a safe distance, we watched in shock. Our friend had pulled over and was walking back to us.

"What happened?" he asked, bewildered.

"No time to figure it out," John said. Then we got into our friend's car and headed for the hospital. I looked back at the burning car. John called the rental agency to let them know what had happened.

We reached the hospital in time where I was once more prepped and wheeled into a surgery room. A catheterization wire was threaded into my arteries to find the blockage so the medicated stent could be placed. To our surprise, there was no blockage. Instead, I was having "coronary spasms" which can feel similar to a blockage and create as much danger as a heart attack. I was given medication to calm my heart and discharged to go home. We stayed a couple of days so I could recover before making the long trip back to Portland and then Spokane.

My disappointment was not that I didn't have a blockage—why would I welcome another stent? But I was baffled at why this was happening. I felt like the women who touched Jesus' garment:

> A large crowd followed and pressed around him. And a woman was there who had been subject to bleeding for twelve years. She had suffered a great deal under the care of many doctors and had spent all she had, yet instead of getting better she grew worse. When she heard about Jesus, she came up behind him in the crowd and touched his cloak, because she thought, "If I just touch his clothes, I will be healed." Immediately her bleeding stopped and she felt in her body that she was freed from her suffering. At once Jesus realized that power had gone out from him. He turned around in the crowd and asked, "Who touched my clothes?"

> You see the people crowding against you, his disciples answered, and yet you can ask, "Who touched me?" But Jesus kept looking around to see who had done it. Then the woman, knowing what had happened to her, came and fell at his feet and, trembling with fear, told him the whole truth. He said to her, "Daughter, your faith has healed you. Go in peace and be freed from your suffering" (Mark 5:25-34 NIV).

I considered these verses and wondered what I was doing wrong. I had pursued one cure after another. My attempts to go to Canada to get a medicated stent ended after I found out their government-funded health care would not accept my insurance. I even contacted a cousin in Italy to find out if the University of Pisa would accept me as a patient. But unfavorable relations with the pharmacological companies in the U.S. had created a bad relationship with Americans. They would not see me.

I chased after not only the doctor in San Diego and his cohort in New York, but also saw the third member of this alliance in Seattle at the University Hospital. He had no more answers for me.

As the woman who touched Jesus' garment, I longed for a way to tap into His healing power. This woman had a seemingly incurable condition. She desperately wanted Jesus to heal her. Sometimes we feel that our problems will keep us from God, we undermine His deity when we doubt His ability to heal us. It is more about when and how He will heal. I may not have seen an answer to my desire to be healed at this time, but later on I would realize His plan was not set to my agenda.

During one of my frequent hospitalizations, I was in the shower getting ready to have yet another nuclear stress test. Exhausted by the constant testing and procedures, I prayed: "Lord, please, either heal me and take away the pain or show the doctors what needs to be done so I can get over this and get on with life."

Immediately, but gently, the Lord replied, "*I cannot heal you until you are ready to accept how I choose to heal you. And I am not finished yet.*"

Those words were gentle yet firm. "But I have prayed that I will accept whatever you choose," I stated with surety. As I pondered my reaction during the week after, I wondered if I had.

Shortly after this word from God, I was faced with His promise. It was 4:00 a.m., and a tall, dark, and bellowing technician came into my room to do an EKG. I always marvel at the timing in a hospital. Just when you sink off into a much-needed reprieve of sleep, someone has to take blood, check your temperature, or do something else nonessential. As he did the EKG, we talked about open-heart surgery. As young as he was, he had survived the surgery just a few years prior and touted how much better he was. "It was the best thing I ever did," he said. "I feel great now."

After he left, I lay there in the solemn shadows and, finally, it made sense. I can't explain what happened. It wasn't a definite thing. But I knew at that moment that God wanted all of me. He is a jealous God and nothing can come between Him and me. Nothing. "Okay, Lord. If you want me to accept however you choose to heal me, I will. I will go into this angioplasty singing!" I called John as soon as it was morning and told him not to worry—I was joyful and happy. Surgery would go fine. Everything was great. I sensed he wasn't as convinced. He, too, was weary.

That morning I was wheeled into the catheterization lab for the angioplasty. I was beaming. The nurses all knew me and had upbeat music playing—'50s music. There was an air of jocularity as the doctor arrived. He obviously wasn't as happy as I felt. I was having chest pain even though being pumped with massive medications. All got quiet as he entered my heart with the catheter. The monitor pulsated with the beating of my heart. This time he searched much longer than before. When he was done, he turned the monitor towards me. There was no blockage to be found! Nothing. All clear! I was so elated. "God healed my arteries!" I told everyone.

John was so happy—everyone was happy. I felt great! The doctor came in later on and suggested antidepressants for my anxiety. "But I'm not anxious," I appealed to him.

"I've been doing this for 13 years," he informed me. "People say they are not anxious but they really are and don't know it. At least the antidepressants will help you sleep."

"But I sleep fine," I continued to protest. "Will antidepressants help my heart?"

"No," he answered.

"Then I refuse them. I don't need them."

Part of "accepting how God healed me" was being humiliated as I was accused of "creating" this last incident. When John confronted the doctor as to why the previous tests showed the blockage, he could only make excuses about reading the results. I had to swallow my pride and face belittlement when I shared how God healed me.

God did heal me, as He would on many occasions. When you pray, ask what you will, but ask without an agenda. Know that God will answer your petition in a perfect way.

After this one procedure, blockages continued to form and more stents and procedures were performed. On one such hospital stay, in February 2002, I was told it had become too dangerous to keep clearing out my main artery. A heart surgeon was called to come in to see me. The first thing he told me was that he was a Christian. The next statement was not as comforting, "Your main artery is about to collapse, and if it does, you will surely die unless you let me perform a double-bypass surgery on you."

I knew as hard as his words were that they were seasoned with skill and wisdom. When John arrived in the room, we agreed to the surgery.

I was readied on a Monday, early in the morning, and brought to the OR. An operation that should have taken three to four hours lasted for six, and although the bypasses were successful, the surgeon told John that they had a lot of trouble with excess internal bleeding. I was now in the cardiac intensive care unit and would be watched carefully.

As the day progressed, the internal bleeding grew worse. After a blood transfusion and attempts to keep me from losing too much blood, my condition became critical. That night, the surgeon told John he had to open me up again and undo all the tremendous work it takes to put someone back together after such a traumatic surgery. He had to find the problem and stop the bleeding. He also cautioned John that the chances my heart would stop from the pressure were great. And if so, I would not survive.

The surgeon stayed with John as I was transported back to surgery and an emergency team was assembled. John was allowed to go as far as the operating room, then he found himself alone in the waiting room. It was terrifying for him. He broke down and prayed for the Lord to help, to comfort, to heal, and to help him understand why this was happening. An hour or so later, the hospital Chaplain and some friends from church arrived. They sat and prayed with him and waited for hours into Tuesday morning.

Finally, the surgeon came out and let everyone know I had made it through. He had found the area causing the massive blood loss. After cleaning everything up and placing more tubes in my chest, I was back in intensive care.

I did not wake up until late Tuesday evening. From then on it was a painfully slow, physically and emotionally difficult recovery. Yet never did I become angry at God. I was distressed and pleaded for Him to spare my family and me this horrific experience, but I was totally willing to go through whatever He had planned for me. I know His purpose is always in my best interest.

While I was in the intensive care unit, John read to me from the Bible. My son Jonathan had sent me a message to read Psalm 86. "It will help you, Mom," he said. "It's about God fighting for you."

The one thing I will keep in my heart are the only words I heard while in a coma. Although I never heard the nurses or the doctors speaking to me, I did hear the precious words "I love you" that John whispered in my ear.

After such a difficult surgery, and the many procedures done to keep me alive and hopefully give me what is often coldly termed as "quality of life," my health continued to degrade. At one point, my medical insurance company assigned me a case manager named Carole.

My first impression at the idea was annoyance. "Oh no they don't! I don't want anyone to report to or explain my problems to." The last thing I wanted was someone else meddling with my appointments and needs.

Clouded by exhaustion and skepticism, I thwarted the efforts of my insurance company and would not answer Carole's phone calls. But her persistence annoyed me, so I decided to finally answer her the next time she called and make it clear that I did not need nor want her help.

If I had any hindsight about how my case manager would play into what happened next, I would never have been so defensive about her contacting me. The instinct to avoid any more aspects of the "process" I was fumbling through, along with the urge to minimize more requirements, caused me to be mistrustful.

But soon after we talked, Carole convinced me to become part of the insurance company's patient care assistance program. She sent me the paperwork and I woefully filled out the forms. We talked once a week and she often helped me with the insurance claims, appointments, and medical concerns.

One day, Carole called about a clinical trial she had discovered on a Website. It was targeted for people who had no more options—their heart disease had progressed past all possible treatments, and open-heart surgery was no longer able to help get blood flow to cardiac muscle. My cardiologist had dubbed my condition a "full metal jacket," as my main coronary artery was completely lined with metal stents. I found myself almost in a vegetative state and so weak I could not even walk to the mailbox in the front of my house.

The trial Carole found was for CardioVascular BioTherapeutic's (a pharmaceutical company in Las Vegas) "Cardio Vascu-Grow," a growth hormone that produces new blood vessel growth around the heart. This new technology was engineered in Germany by Dr. Thomas Stegmann and it was already changing the lives of many people in his country. I immediately got online and read the requirements for the trial and presented the info to my cardiologist. He felt I was a perfect candidate and we began the application process.

The paperwork and medical testing to see if I was eligible was extensive, but the day grew closer when I would travel to Penn State Milton S. Hershey Medical Center in Hershey, Pennsylvania for the surgery and treatment. The operation was scheduled for December and the local newspaper printed a story about me titled "She needs a Christmas Miracle."

> A day without heart problems is almost unthinkable for the 43-year-old Spokane Valley woman. She spends much of her day sedated on a couch because the excitement of everyday life is too much. Her kitchen counter resembles a small pharmacy.

> But Scinto is not taking her cardiac problems lying down. Two months ago when doctors told her they had tried everything, the mother from Greenacres got on the Internet and enrolled in an experimental cloned gene program in Hershey, Pennsylvania.
>
> Scinto said the procedure is her Christmas miracle. Her Spokane cardiologist, Donald Canaday, considers the experimental procedure a final alternative.
>
> "The reason we got her into gene therapy is because it is the only thing that hasn't been done," Canaday said.
>
> "We are just so grateful for this holiday miracle," Scinto said. "Even though we will spend Christmas and New Years alone in Pennsylvania, we are just happy that I may get some strength and health back."[16]

Traveling to Hershey was difficult and I arrived there in a wheelchair, unable to walk on my own without the fear of a looming heart attack. But a week after the FGF-1 was injected into my heart, I was walking a mile a day. Five weeks later I traveled home and effortlessly carted in wood for our fireplace and shoveled six inches of snow from our driveway! The news was out that it was a 100 percent turnaround and one of the headlines in the Central Pennsylvania Business Journal read "SHE'S TOO WELL!"

> "This looks beautiful," Boehmer said about the images from Scinto's last heart X-ray. Iodine — the dark liquid that illuminates blood flow on an X-ray — shot freely through her artery and venal bypass. He grinned.
>
> "Aw, man…can't beat that," Boehmer said.

> The X-rays showed a vessel had sprouted and formed a loop around a blockage in her artery, sparing Scinto from a heart attack. Another vessel appears to have restored blood flow to a bypass that had become blocked. Her stress test was normal. "This is the point in clinical care when we usually claim victory," Boehmer said from the office at Penn State Milton S. Hershey Medical Center.
>
> Scinto had improved so much by that June 7 visit that she would no longer be eligible for her experimental treatment, which is being reviewed by the U.S. Food and Drug Administration. In December, doctors at Hershey injected a synthetic protein into her heart.
>
> "Right now, she's too well," Boehmer said."[17]

The FGF-1 injection gave me my life back! Within four to five days, this miraculous growth hormone grew new coronary vessels around my failing heart. There were no side effects, no health issues—just a chance to live again!

Dr. Stegmann, professor of surgery and a world renowned cardiovascular surgeon, began researching the potential of angiogenesis in Germany in the early nineties. His work led to the first clinical trials of the FGF-1 growth hormone in the United States of which I was a part in 2003. Dr. Stegmann expresses his own experience after hearing of my story:

> Under normal circumstances, a physician always sees his patient after surgery. He or she takes time to discuss how the surgery went with the patient's family and loved ones. This practice was implemented so long ago that it is hard to say when it came to pass. What is strange for me is that a patient I did not even know

went through my US clinical trial, using a procedure I pioneered.

I had no idea how great her suffering really was. When I started my own clinical trials in Germany, I knew the patients—most of them were well over fifty years old and after the procedure, I was able to talk with all of them. They all were diagnosed with Acute Coronary Heart Disease and had reached the point of "No Option" or "Zero Option" meaning additional coronary artery stents or bypass surgery would not help get blood and oxygen back into their hearts. Most of them truly had about two years left to live.

I knew our protein therapy worked and was not surprised to hear of its success, but listening to the story of such a young woman, only in her forties and just starting her life, and learning that my discovery kept her alive, somehow at that particular moment struck me as one of the most profound moments in my own life. Right there and then it clearly awakened within my mind the reality of my purpose. Here I was, sitting and quietly observing this woman when just like opening your eyes to a new day, I understood that everything I have been fighting for, all with the hopes of finding a way to stop the unnecessary suffering, finally was happening. This therapy worked and did actually take the pain and suffering away from those in misery due to heart disease, and although it was not a cure, it can help those in need.

To actually meet this woman who has gone through so much, as she stood in front of me with her one desire, to shake my hand, the hand of the man she claims saved her life was overwhelming and heartfelt to me. Even after all the years of being a heart surgeon, knowing that

> I finally found the way to help stop the pain, allowing people like Cindy to get back to her life and try to have some normalcy that so many of us take for granted, made it one of the most wonderful days of my life.[18]

As I recount this experimental procedure and how it came to pass, I think of my hesitancy when I first got news of a case manager becoming part of my life. How tragic the thought that if I had not had the experimental surgery—only the third person in the United States to have it done—I would probably not lived long enough to receive a heart transplant in July 2005.

Although the procedure did not allow me a complete recovery, it was a part of two miracles in my journey. Three months after the experimental injection of FGF-1, another massive blockage was found in my main coronary artery that would have caused a fatal heart attack if the new vessels were not there. And of course, the new vessels brought much needed blood flow to my heart, allowing me to live long enough to wait for a donor heart to be available.

So often after each procedure or surgery, I would chase the dream that I was going to recover completely. Alone one day, I cried and pleaded with God, "Please heal me so I can serve you once again." For years before my illness, I was part of many events at church. I scurried from one area to the next, from changing diapers in the nursery to playing flute on the worship team. I wanted it all back.

God's reply was precise: "You *are* serving me."

I just had to rediscover where it was that God wanted me to be and how He wanted me to serve Him. Chasing a healing, pushing for answers to prayers I "demanded" instead of "presented" to God, would only rob me of His will for my life.

Joni Eareckson Tada, in her book *Joni*, prayed a similar prayer:

> Lord, I know now that You have something planned for my life. But I need help understanding Your will. I need help in knowing Your Word. Please, God, do something in my life to help me serve You and know Your Word.[19]

Joni's prayer was answered. Although she too chased avenues to regain the ability to walk and desired for God to heal her, she found much more to her life through what He provided in place of the losses she had suffered.

In the book of Jeremiah, chapter 36, we read about King Jehoiakim and how he burned the scrolls containing the words of God that Jeremiah and Baruch so painstakingly inscribed. But the word of the Lord came to Jeremiah and in verse 28 we read: "Take another scroll and write on it all the words that were on the first scroll, which Jehoiakim king of Judah burned up." Jeremiah did this and more: "So Jeremiah took another scroll and gave it to the scribe Baruch son of Neriah, and as Jeremiah dictated, Baruch wrote on it all the words of the scroll that Jehoiakim king of Judah had burned in the fire. And many similar words were added to them" (Jeremiah 36:32) NIV.

Jill Briscoe poses this poignant question about Jeremiah and Baruch:

> Would they have faith enough to finish? How would they respond to the voice of God? How would you have responded? Would you start all over again, or would you quit? . . . Jeremiah handed Baruch another scroll and began all over again. They did it again. Yes, they did it again! Now that's faithfulness![20]

Years of work were erased by fire and an evil king, yet Jeremiah and Baruch were willing to not only start over, but to go even further. Chasing the wind can be futile or it can lead us to press on. Make God the wind you press into, and He will hold you up to continue your life as He planned it for you. There is much more ahead.

3 CHAPTER 3
ISN'T IT AMAZING?

Isn't It Amazing

Isn't it amazing what a prayer can do,
When it all seems hopeless it'll pull you through.
Isn't it amazing how a broken heart grows strong,
When every now and then that
Someone special comes along.

I was rolled into the operating room of the heart catheterization lab where a staff was waiting to hook me up to equipment and medications. Big, bad "Dave" came to the holding area to get me. "When I saw 'Cindy Scinto' on the schedule, I had to come get you myself," he commanded. "Why are you here?" His expression was serious—not gruff and comical like it normally was. This was heart catheterization number 34 and Dave was the attending nurse for most of them. Normally, he was known for his attempts at not smiling but I was one patient who could normally coax him into a mischievous grin.

"Is Carol here?" I asked. "Don't take it personally," I assured one of the nurses, "I just love Carol."

"Carol's here," answered Dave. "In fact, she changed her shift so she could be here for you." Carol was another nurse who had attended most of my heart procedures. Her wispy blonde hair, bright eyes, and broad smile always comforted me amid the operating room busyness before I was put to sleep. Her calming hand stroked my forehead as I was lulled off by the anesthesia. It was her concern and comforting presence that I saw last and it stayed with me when I woke up.

Once a year, in July, I have to go through testing and a heart catheterization to be sure my donor heart is doing okay. But here I was in May, having a procedure to see if I really had a blockage in one of the vessels on the left side of my heart. For a few weeks, I had been having chest pain and fatigue. A nuclear stress test a few days prior showed decreased blood flow on the left side and for a transplant of barely three years that is bad news. If the vessels around my heart were already starting to block up, it could mean whatever was originally wrong with me had started to attack this new heart.

I had emailed all the prayer warriors on my email list the night before and asked everyone to pray for a miracle. I asked them to pray it was a fluke and there really was no blockage. With the symptoms I was having and a positive nuclear stress test, the odds of not having a blockage were slim and, short of a miracle, I would be facing some discouraging news.

I also called Charlotte, my heart donor's mom, the night before, "Charlotte, I have to have a heart catheterization. It looks like I may have a blockage in one of the vessels. But don't worry, Charlotte, I am going to tell the doctor to make sure he takes care of Danielle's heart. I won't let anything happen to 'our' heart." Charlotte assured me she would be praying. We were in this together. She lost her daughter to a tragic accident—but I gained a new chance at life through her daughter's act of kindness as an organ donor. (Read about my heart donor and her family in chapter 7.)

The last words I spoke before my eyes shut were to my cardiologist performing the procedure: "Dr. Canaday, you'd better take care of this heart! It's been through enough. Let's make Danielle proud!"

I awoke from the anesthesia back in my room to good news. No blockage! Although the heart had an area of stiffness and elevated pressure, there was *no blockage*. The stiffness is common for a heart that has been damaged, repaired, placed on ice, and then transplanted into another person. Medication was prescribed and more time in my garden was suggested. I knew God healed me. I knew God heard the prayers of many and healed the blockage. Some of the hospital personnel explained it away as an inaccurate test result, but I wouldn't let anyone steal the miracle God performed! In fact, one of my doctors and my heart transplant nurse/coordinator attested the results to a healing from God. Healing is a controversial subject for many, and for some it's an outright impossibility. But I knew God healed my heart.

Many people have heard about *healing*. The subject can either spur someone on to seek God's will or it can become a catalyst for heated arguments. Often, people are made to feel inadequate if the healing they pray for does not come. Some consider it an issue of faith. Personally, I have my own beliefs about healing, but choose not to instigate debate. Instead, I would like to travel the route of healing and answered prayer that has been an integral part of my life.

I remember the first time I experienced a healing from the Lord. Not that miracles hadn't already happened in the two years since becoming a Christian, but this one was a vivid example of the character of God.

I was at a Sunday evening church service at a local park. We had an outdoor service once a month to take church out to the people whom normally didn't come to a church building. I stood in the back of the group during worship service, crutches holding me up. My right foot had a heel spur that was going to have to be surgically removed. It was scheduled for the next Wednesday and I dreaded it.

A woman from the church came over to me and offered to pray with me. "Can I pray for your foot?" she asked.

"Sure," I said, thinking she would just stand there and pray for me.

"No, I want to lay my hands on your feet," she gestured.

Being my silly self, I answered, "Great! While you're down there—how about a massage?" She knelt down, laid her hands on my feet, and began to pray quietly. Within a few minutes I felt a warm sensation go up my leg and a stinging pain in my foot.

Then I heard words spoken to me that weren't really audible; they seemed to be audible, but I can't explain how they sounded. I just knew it was God. "I will be your surgeon."

That was it. I placed my foot down flat on the ground and began to walk without the crutches. There was no more pain. My foot was fine. My foot was healed!

I cancelled my surgery and that week I went to the doctor's office and showed him my foot. I told him God healed it. He had a hard time believing me and even insisted I find another podiatrist.

Who healed my foot? *God.*

Was it the lady who prayed for me, or a faith choice I made? I don't have definitive answers. I don't even want to try to figure it out or come up with a theory. All I know is at that time, in that park, God chose to heal me.

Many Sundays, because of my illness, John and I would attend "virtual church" as I like to call it. We could worship and listen to good teaching from a church locally or back on the East Coast—right in our living room. The Internet makes for a wonderful resource when you are homebound. Many churches have live, online services. One Sunday at home, we were watching our pastor from our church back in Tempe, Arizona and he knew we were logged on so he prayed for me! Technology is amazing!

One morning, while watching Pastor Lloyd Pulley of Calvary Chapel Old Bridge, New Jersey, he shared a quote from a woman in the church who had used the text in her family newsletter. As I listened, I realized that a physical healing isn't always God's priority. What we may think is good for us physically can actually hinder us spiritually.

> I don't understand why sometimes there is a miraculous healing granted while other times there are unanswered prayers to healing. Sometimes God's no to our prayers can mean a yes to something greater in our heart. My question is this: What is more of a miracle—a healed body or a changed heart? Our bodies are just temporary, but our hearts and souls count for eternity. Changed hearts require our permission for the working of grace in our lives. God never forces us to change."[22]

This wisdom comes from a woman who has seen much suffering as she watches her husband hold on and fight for his life. A physical healing or a changed heart—which do you think will bring about more strength in a person? Which do you think will have lasting benefits?

One day I met a girlfriend at the grocery store. I was wheeling myself around with my broken leg (see chapter 8). We chatted for a while and she exclaimed her disbelief that I had yet another physical hurdle to tackle. As many people do, she told me how much of an encouragement I always was for her. But the story she shared next, reminded me of the incredible care God has for us. Only a week before, Mindy had been hit by a train! And here she was proclaiming God's miraculous answer to prayer.

At her weekly Bible Study, Mindy shared how she felt like she always got along okay as a Christian, but had never seen the power of God really evident in her life. She wanted more. She wanted to experience God's sovereignty firsthand. So she prayed that night for God to reveal himself to her in a very real way.

The next day, she was on her way home with her two grandchildren in her vehicle. There was a railroad crossing before the turnoff to her house. As was customary when they come to this train crossing, Mindy asked her granddaughter Ally, "Is there a train coming?"

"No, Grandma," chimes Ally. Mindy had already looked and did not see a train. She began to cross the tracks and out of nowhere, a train appeared not 100 feet from the crossing.

Mindy knew they would be hit if she didn't get off the tracks. Reacting with fear as the adrenaline shot through her body, she *thought* she floored the gas to take off, but instead found her vehicle in park. The train blew its horn as it passed in front of Mindy's eyes. The blur of the cars from the train was interrupted by the sight of her bumper flying down the tracks.

Ally pleaded furiously, "Grandma, back up."

Mindy put her vehicle in reverse as the train began to slow down. She turned to look at the kids and they were fine. They weren't even crying. She reassured them that God was in their car and they were going to be okay.

In reality, Mindy's vehicle should have been pushed along with the train and possibly smashed, injuring her and her two grandchildren. Instead, the train "seared" the front of her vehicle right down to the radiator. The car never budged. It remained in park, running, and it was as if the train simply "cut" a slice off the front. This was physically impossible!

Mindy was fine, the kids were fine, and she stood there in shock thinking, "We just got hit by a train, and we are fine."

Getting a ride from a friend, Mindy went to pick up her other granddaughter, Sophie, from day care. Dazed at the moment, she clutched Sophie's take home papers from her school basket and stuffed them in her purse. That evening, when everyone was gone, she was thinking about the day and wondering why God had saved them.

God answered Mindy; "I pulled Sophie's papers out of my purse to see what she had taken home and there was her week's memory verse; 'For by grace you have been saved through faith; and that not of yourselves, it is the gift of God' (Ephesians 2:8 NASB).

"I cried and knew God had answered my request."

God answered her prayer from the night before. She asked Him to show her His power in her life. God knew this "accident" would happen and He not only saved them from disaster but also used this to display His love, care, protection, and compassion for Mindy. "For by grace you have been saved…"

Prayer, persistence, and the power of God—we pray for help, we are persistent in faith, and we must grab from the power of God.

Have you ever read stories of a duck or a goose surviving and living with an arrow shot through its body? It's a strange story to hear about and even more interesting is how *often* you hear it reported.

Here is one such story from *The Yuma Sun* newspaper in Yuma, Arizona.

> Duck shot by arrow is recovering, by Nicole E. Squibbs
>
> A local veterinarian is treating the mallard duck that was swimming with an arrow protruding from its

> body and was rescued by Yuma Fire Department from the canal near 1st Street and Avenue A.
>
> She said the arrow entered the duck above the right armpit and exited below the left armpit, puncturing her lungs and air sacs.
>
> "I haven't actually seen an arrow sticking out of a bird that is still alive, ever," Haugo said. "I thought, 'Oh my God,' but she is so darn lucky about this arrow... God was watching out for her."
>
> Haugo said the arrow "just missed the really important stuff," such as the heart and spine.
>
> She said the duck will not be able to return to the wild due to a fractured wing from the incident. "She will never be able to fly again."
>
> Currently, the duck is in rehab at Haugo's home, where she's had up to 30 ducks at one time. The recent addition makes a current total of five.
>
> It is unclear if she has any mortal injuries. For the most part, she is doing pretty good. [23]

This duck was persistent but even the veterinarian had to give God the credit. How often do we encounter times in our lives where we feel we are going through each day with an arrow through our souls? Days when we want to fall away and stop the world around us from spinning with tornado strength?

Isn't it amazing what a prayer can do?

Only a few months after my first heart attack, my sister Annie was determined to get me in to see a cardiologist in New York City who was spearheading the trials for medicated heart stents. Dr. Jeffrey Moses was representing Johnson and Johnson Company as they worked to get FDA approval for tiny, coiled, metal stents with medication on them. These types of stents, once placed in a coronary vessel cleared of a blockage, would prevent—the forming of a blockage within a stent.

All the stents placed in my heart were continuously blocking back up, making it very dangerous. Each time they blocked back up, my cardiologist had to go in and "rotablade" the interior of the stent. Each time he did this, it thinned the wall of my arteries, even more.

My sister saw a show on the morning news about Dr. Moses. She called me about it and told me she wanted to speak directly to himand ask him to allow me to travel to New York to see him personally.

"You're crazy!" was my baffled reply. "He's famous. You won't get past the receptionist!"

After my sister hung up with me she placed her hand on her phone and prayed for the Lord to do a miracle and let her get through. Then she placed the call.

"Dr. Jeffrey Moses' office," The receptionist answered.

"Can I speak to Dr. Moses?" my sister asked.

"Certainly, hold on a moment."

Within a few seconds, Dr. Moses himself got on the phone! Annie was amazed. She composed herself and told him my predicament. He instructed her to have me send him my records and a CD with films from my last heart catheterization.

By August 26, 2002, I was in Lennox Hill Hospital in Manhattan where Dr. Moses performed a heart angioplasty on me. He not only placed two new stents in my vessels, but he was determined to clear the 100 percent blockage in my LAD—Left Anterior Descending artery. This is the most important vessel and mine was completely blocked.

I remember starting to wake up towards the end of the procedure. Here was Dr. Moses, draped over my body, twisting the wire tubing that was threaded up to my heart. He was fiercely trying to clear the LAD. As he worked to free it, he yelled, "Come on, come on, let me at you!" His wiry hair was tossed back and his face tensed with determination.

Finally, the blockage was cleared and blood began to flow. Everyone in the operating room was clapping!

While I was in recovery, I asked one of the nurses about his performance. She replied, "Oh that's Dr. Moses. He's known as 'The Cowboy'!"

Not even a year later, back in my home in Spokane, Washington, my main bypass (I had a double-bypass, open-heart surgery in February of 2002) sustained a blockage right where it was connected to my LAD. If Dr. Moses had not cleared out the blockage, I would have certainly suffered a fatal heart attack. This was a prayer answered with many blessings attached!

Pray with expectation, not an agenda!

Earlier, when I was fighting for an opportunity to be part of the experimental surgery in Hershey, Pennsylvania, there were copious amounts of hurdles to overcome through the approval process before I was even accepted into the clinical trial. My cardiologist at home was directed to perform all sorts of testing to be sure I met all the requirements for not only the efficacy of the drug, but also to be sure I would not suffer any undue complications from possible side effects.

As everyone in the medical community wanted me to have this opportunity, the evaluation was tempered with deep emotions and sighs of relief every time as I got past each requirement. A lot of prayer and many miracles happened on a regular basis. But once I traveled to Hershey, I had to go through another battery of tests before the actual surgery date.

Only three days into the final testing at the Milton S. Hershey Medical Center in Hershey, I received a sobering phone call at my hotel. Something in one of the requirements failed to match what had been done back home at my local doctor's office. I was going to be disqualified for the program.

I sunk into the ratty mattress in my shabby hotel room and let out a sigh of defeat. *Oh Lord, please don't send me back to Spokane to die. Why would I get this far only to be turned down? Please, Lord, make it work out.* I prayed silently to myself and then waited for the nurse to call me back with a final decision. I was preparing myself for the worst news.

Almost two hours later, my cell phone rang. The number on the display indicated it was from the hospital. I could actually see the building from my hotel window so I walked over to peer out in the distance as I spoke with the nurse.

"Well, we finished our evaluation and decided after all the testing was properly weighed, you will make the criteria for the clinical trial by the smallest margin. Be here tomorrow by 9:00 a.m. for your surgery pre-op work-up. And by the way—congratulations!"

I was stunned. A few hours before I was facing defeat and possible death and now my life was once more presented to me as a token prize. How many times in a week or a day could I have life and death paraded before me?

Of course, the trial worked and played an enormous part in me being alive today.

Isn't it amazing?

From near miss heart attacks, to experimental surgeries, I never knew what was going to happen to me when I woke up each day. I never knew what other miracle would keep me alive. One of the miracles that kept me alive was a very small device I became very dependent on.

By December of 2002, pressure and problems with my heart caused it to work hard to stay rhythmic. At one point, there were so many PVCs (premature ventricular contractions–see Glossary on page 195 for definition.) that I needed to have an ablation to calm things down. This is a procedure in which a specialized cardiologist—called an electrophysiological cardiologist who deals with abnormalities in the electrical system of the heart—goes in through a catheterization and uses a laser to disengage the extra electrical pathways that are causing the heart to have abnormal heartbeats. I was informed that the procedure could cause too much of the electrical system to be destroyed and leave me with a heartbeat that is too slow. If so, I would need a pacemaker implanted to keep my heart at the proper heart rate.

Of course, as things seemed to go for me, I woke up with a pacemaker implanted in my left shoulder. Again, I was just happy to have gotten through the surgery well and looked forward to once again trying to go home a "rehabilitate."

Time went by and I became accustomed to the regular pacemaker checkups. I must admit however, even though I had gained much compassion for elderly heart disease patients, I found it discouraging to sit in the waiting room for my pacemaker check with the rest of the patients. Although I was often told many young people also had heart disease hurdles, I always seemed to be the only young person in the waiting room.

One time I went in for my checkup and told the technician I was feeling very *off*. My heart seemed to be hanging at exactly 80 bpm and I was often dizzy, weak and especially worn-out.

Once the technician hooked me up to the diagnostic computer, she ran a few tests and asked me to wait until she got back with the doctor. My cardiologist came in after a few minutes and was surprised to see me sitting up.

"How do you feel?" he asked cautiously.

"Well, weak and funny," I answered. "What is going on?"

He answered me with a tone of disbelief. "Your pacemaker is now running at 100 percent. In other words, your heart has completely stopped beating on its own and is entirely dependent on the pacemaker. You are now 'pacemaker dependent' and your heart will never beat on its own again."

I was once again amazed at another miracle. If I had not needed an ablation and had a pacemaker implanted, my heart would have stopped beating and I would have been dead before I even landed on the ground. "Pacemaker dependent" meant that the security check at the airport, a highly sensitive security sensor at a department store, or any other electromagnetic field could stop my pacemaker and kill me instantly. The news was leading me into a whole new other way of living, but at least I was alive—again.

Prayer is answered every time we petition God for help. It may not be the way we intend or hope for, but the answers from God are never the wrong ones.

In April of 2005, one week before I had the near death experience in the ER, I was driving my son Jonathan to a doctor's appointment. He was 15 and just getting excited about starting to drive. My husband had already let him drive our old truck in a field to get him accustomed to handling a vehicle larger than his dirt bike.

We were on the freeway, doing 60 miles an hour, when I began to feel dizzy. Within a few minutes, my legs and feet became numb and also the left side of my face. I feared I was having a stroke. I couldn't feel the gas pedal or brakes and had to quickly decide what to do. I prayed a hurried prayer that God would sustain me until I could exit the freeway. It was too dangerous to stop abruptly.

Looking over at Jonathan, I merely asked him how he felt about driving if he had to. He looked at me with a pale face. Instead of jumping at the chance, he was worried. He knew something was very wrong.

I prayed once more and asked the Lord to get us to the hospital safely. I am sure angels took over where my feet and legs could no longer operate the gas and brakes. We made it to the front of the hospital but I was not able to function well enough to get us to the ER around back.

When I stepped out of my van, my knees gave way from under me and I collapsed to the ground. Holding myself up by the door, I asked Jonathan to go in and get a wheelchair for me. He came back with the wheelchair and brought it around to where I was holding myself up.

"Mom, I would have been here sooner, but the lady at the desk thought I was trying to steal the wheelchair. She made me give her my phone number. I tried to tell her it was for you." Jonathan was frantic by now.

"Don't worry. Do you know how to get to the ER?" I asked, more scared for him than myself. He had to be terrified and now he had the responsibility of getting me to the ER which was far from the front entrance to the hospital.

"I know where it is, Mom." Although only 15, Jonathan took control of the situation and began wheeling me into the hospital and down the myriad of hallways. He was pushing the wheelchair so fast I could feel the cool hospital air brush against my hot cheeks.

He got me to the ER and I called my friend Terry to pick him up. My husband was out of town for work, and there was no one at home. I didn't want Jonathan to have to be there with me and I didn't want him to go home alone.

Terry picked him up with her husband and she stayed with me. My heart had gone into an episode of tachycardia—rapid heartbeat. This had happened to me before, but this time it lasted so long that I was near a heart attack. The nurses in the ER worked furiously to get my heart rate down and, after a couple of hours, it finally subsided. I was admitted and stayed for a week, only to be admitted again one day after going home. (This was the story I wrote about in chapter 1 when I came in by ambulance and actually had an experience with dying.)

It was a miracle I could drive long enough to safely get us to the hospital and it was a miracle I didn't have a heart attack right then, possibly causing an accident and hurting Jonathan and me or someone else. Isn't it amazing!

Many times I prayed and asked the Lord to do another miracle. He answered so many prayers, and yet every time one was answered, another life-threatening need would arise.

King David, in Psalm 6, wrote about deliverance from God while in deep troubled times. In verse 2, he pleads for God to heal him: "Be merciful to me, Lord, for I am faint; O Lord, heal me, for my bones are in agony" (NIV). And then in verse 9, David shows the answer from God after a cascading psalm of despair, "The Lord has heard my cry for mercy; the Lord accepts my prayer" (NIV).

Jeremiah, in the Old Testament, makes a parallel statement: "Heal me, O Lord, and I shall be healed; save me, and I shall be saved: for thou art my praise" (Jeremiah 17:14 KJV).

I remember looking for God to answer my prayer for healing when I was very young. When I was ten years old, I developed diabetes. Not only was it traumatic for my mom, family, and myself, but 34 years ago there was a lot less known about how to treat and live with diabetes. At that time, my family was part of a traditional church in New York. Each Sunday one of the standard responses in the mass would be, "Only say the words, and I shall be healed" (see Matthew 8:8b NASB).

Every time I repeated this response, I would take a deep breath and wait for a moment, hoping God would heal me of diabetes. But the healing never came. Not truly knowing Jesus, I couldn't understand why He did not heal me.

After becoming chronically ill with life-threatening heart disease, I found myself again pleading with the Lord for healing. But each time I prayed, I prayed with an *agenda*, wanting the healing to come in my own way and my own timing.

It was like the day I cried out to God, "Lord, why haven't You healed me?"

His gentle reply was: "I cannot heal you until you are ready to accept how I choose to heal you. And I am not finished yet."

I can still feel the power of His response and after He spoke these words to me, I began to see all the ways He was answering prayer—maybe not by my design but definitely by His design.

Divine healing cannot be defined by Webster's Dictionary nor can it be forced by our will. The answer for healing may not come until God's appointed time. Or the healing may be so different than what we prayed for that we might not recognize it as a healing. God's purpose for healing cannot be limited by our personal desires. The strength we gain by trusting Him to take us through our trials sets an example for others who may be suffering and in need of encouragement.

In his book, *A Shepherd Looks at Psalm 23*, Phillip Keller uses his firsthand experience as a sheep rancher to take a unique look at this well known psalm. He emphasizes the encouragement a Christian can be to others when they accept the "Shepherd's" provision as they "walk through the valley of the shadow of death."

> It is a most reassuring and reinforcing experience to the child of God to discover that there is, even in the dark valley, a source of strength and courage to be found in God. Storms may break about me, predators may attack, the rivers of reverses may threaten to inundate me. But because He is in the situation with me, I shall not fear. The person with a powerful confidence in Christ; the one who has proved by past experience that God is with him in adversity; the one who walks through life's dark valleys without fear, his head held high, is the one who in turn is a tower of strength and a source of inspiration to his companions.[24]

Healing, or "the process of getting well," comes when we realize God has a specific purpose for each of our lives. When we accept how He chooses to heal us, we then gain new strength not only for ourselves but for those God puts in our path.

Many times throughout my years of illness, friends, acquaintances, and even perfect strangers have offered me, with sincerity, ways to *get healed*. And they still do as I continue to persevere through chronic illnesses. I know they are all looking out for me and have only the best intentions, but the offers always have a formula whether it comes in a natural remedy, a product, a new discovery, a spiritual theory, or even a healer or place of healing to attend.

Recently, I met a sweet woman for the first time at a seminar. After laughing about my troublesome health issues, she began to tell me about a building that housed a healing center. She was positive that if I went there, God would heal me. I am sure there are some dynamic prayer warriors with this organization, but my reply shocked her and left her without a defense to answer to me. I used the wisdom from Cindy Mah whom I quoted earlier in this chapter.

"I appreciate your concern, but what is more powerful—a physical healing or a changed heart? God is using me even in my weakness. I am sharing with so many people who are being encouraged by the absolute power of God in my life. If I were to be healed, I would be done. Oh, I would still have my story to tell, but by living it out each day, I can be a very real example of faithful perseverance."

She smiled at me and pondered my answer. I know some of the people who offer me solutions for my tragic health problems are wondering about why I—or they even—pray anymore. Some people have come to a point of crisis in their view of prayer as I continue to reach more milestones of despairing health concerns rather than triumphant victories of powerful prayer.

In his seasoned wisdom, Nick Vujicic of Australia illustrates his acceptance of God's will for his life. Nick was born without arms and legs, yet he now ministers to people all over the globe. Here is his idea of victorious living:

> Circumstances do not have to change for you to become victorious. It is our hearts that need to be filled with the Holy Spirit.[25]

He writes this message on the front page of his Website to encourage all people:

> God has used me to let people know in countless schools, churches, prisons, orphanages, hospitals, stadiums and in face-to-face encounters with individuals how very precious they are to God. Secondly, it's my pleasure to assure them that God does have a plan for their lives that is purposeful. For God took my life, one that others might disregard as having any significance and filled me with His purpose and showed me His plans to move hearts and lives toward Him. Understanding this, though faced with struggles, you can overcome too.[26]

So why does it seem that we pray and sometimes, although we may believe God always answer our prayers, our request fails to eventuate? I have found, through trial, study, and prayer, that prayer is not only to receive an answer. Below is a list of the main reasons we pray:

Nine Reasons We Pray:

1. *God is close to us or near to us*: "What other nation is so great as to have their gods near them the way the LORD our God is near us whenever we pray to him?" (Deuteronomy 4:7 NIV).

2. *God rewards us*: "And when you pray, you shall not be like the hypocrites. For they love to pray standing in the synagogues and on the corners of the streets, that they may be seen by men. Assuredly, I say to you, they have their reward. But you, when you pray, go into your room, and when you have shut your door, pray to your Father who is in the secret place; and your Father who sees in secret will reward you openly" (Matthew 6:5-6 NKJV).

3. *Not to fall into temptation*: "Then He said to them, 'My soul is exceedingly sorrowful, even to death. Stay here and watch with Me.' He went a little farther and fell on His face, and prayed, saying, 'O My Father, if it is possible, let this cup pass from Me; nevertheless, not as I will, but as You will.' Then He came to the disciples and found them sleeping, and said to Peter, 'What! Could you not watch with Me one hour? Watch and pray, lest you enter into temptation. The spirit indeed is willing, but the flesh is weak' " (Matthew 26:38-41 NKJV).

4. *God wants us to*: "But I say to you who hear: Love your enemies, do good to those who hate you, bless those who curse you, and pray for those who spitefully use you. To him who strikes you on the one cheek, offer the other also. And from him who takes away your cloak, do not withhold your tunic either. Give to everyone who asks of you. And from him who takes away your goods do not ask them back. And just as you want men to do to you, you also do to them likewise" (Luke 6:27-30 NIV).

5. *To be made well or healed*: "Is anyone among you suffering? Let him pray. Is anyone cheerful? Let him sing psalms. Is anyone among you sick? Let him call for the elders of the church, and let them pray over him, anointing him with oil in the name of the LORD. And the prayer of faith will save the sick, and the LORD will raise him up. And if he has committed sins, he will be forgiven. Confess your trespasses to one another, and pray for one another, that you may be healed. The effective, fervent prayer of a righteous man avails much. Elijah was a man with a nature like ours, and he prayed earnestly that it would not rain; and it did not rain on the land for three years and six months. And he prayed again, and the heaven gave rain, and the earth produced its fruit" (James 5:13-18 NKJV).

6. *So God can hear us*: "Then the priests, the Levites, arose and blessed the people, and their voice was heard; and their prayer came up to His holy dwelling place, to heaven" (2 Chronicles 30: 27 NKJV). "The LORD has heard my supplication; The LORD will receive my prayer" (Psalms 6:9 NKJV). "I call on you, O God, for you will answer me; give ear to me and hear my prayer" (Psalms 17:6 NIV).

7. *To please God; to make God happy*: "The LORD detests the sacrifice of the wicked, but the prayer of the upright pleases him" (Proverbs 15:8 NIV).

8. *To receive an answer*: "Therefore I say to you, whatever things you ask when you pray, believe that you receive them, and you will have them" (Mark 11:24 NKJV).

9. *To recieve peace from God*: "Be anxious for nothing, but in everything by prayer and supplication, with thanksgiving, let your requests be made known to God; and the peace of God, which

surpasses all understanding, will guard your hearts and minds through Christ Jesus" (Philippians 4:6-7 NKJV).

Pray without an *agenda*. Pray without *ceasing*. Pray knowing God will answer in *His own way*, but for *your own good*. Then, when the miracles do come, don't doubt that God is the author. Too often a miracle comes from persistent prayer and the petitioner may not accept the very miracle they prayed for.

Witnesses to a miracle either see the power of God or deny what they know could not be physically possible. Consider the Israelites who had already witnessed many miracles of God: "They refused to listen and failed to remember the miracles you performed among them. . . But you are a forgiving God, gracious and compassionate, slow to anger and abounding in love. Therefore you did not desert them . . ." (Nehemiah 9:17 NIV). How easily they forgot and turned from Him. What are miracles and what is their purpose? Bible scholar M.G. Easton M.A., D.D. says:

> Miracles are seals of a divine mission. The sacred writers appealed to them as proofs that they were messengers of God. Our Lord also appealed to miracles as a conclusive proof of his divine mission (John 5: 20,36; 10:25,38). Where miracles are there certainly God is. Unbelievers deny that any testimony can prove a miracle, because they say miracles are impossible. An atheist or a pantheist must, as a matter of course, deny the possibility of miracles; but to one who believes in a personal God, who in his wisdom may see fit to interfere with the ordinary processes of nature, miracles are not impossible, nor are they incredible.[27]

Although an atheist must deny the existence of miracles, like the Israelites who turned their backs on God, it is not that they can explain them away, just that they choose to ignore what they know to be true. The only time a miracle should be ignored is if it is counterfeit; that is, having at least two distinguishing characteristics. One test is if the miracle is not really supernatural in nature but merely a matter of slight of hand or some other sort of trickery or illusion. The other test—does it lead you to Jesus? Does it come from God? (See 2 Thessalonians, chapter 2.)

Miracles also demonstrate God's bountiful love for people. David Wilkerson illustrates this point in his monthly newsletter,

> As we search through the Gospel accounts, we're struck by the number of times Jesus performed miracles but instructed the people, "Do not tell anyone about this. Don't let this news be spread abroad." After healing two blind men, Christ told the men to keep the miracle to themselves. "Jesus straitly charged them, saying, See that no man know it" Matthew 9:30 You see, Jesus didn't want the people following Him for His miracles. He wanted their devotion because His tender words captured their hearts.[28]

In the psalms, King David comes very close to seeing God as being without mercy when so much tribulation came upon him. "I cried out to God for help; I cried out to God to hear me. When I was in distress, I sought the LORD; Has God forgotten to be merciful? I will remember the deeds of the LORD; yes, I will remember your miracles of long ago. I will meditate on all your works and consider all your mighty deeds" (Psalm 77:1,2,9,11, 12 NIV).

David stopped himself and took a look back at all God had done in his life. A miracle is the response of a yielded heart. A person's heart must also be surrendered to God to either perform a miracle or attest to one. David yielded his heart to God.

How many times has God performed miracles for us to see and know He is real, and yet in times of trouble, we easily forget and fall into despair? No matter how many miracles we witness, it should only take one to build our faith. Where miracles occur, God is there!

Tim Hansel is the founder of Summit Expedition, a wilderness survival school for individuals seeking deeper experiences with themselves, others, and God. For years he has lived with continual physical pain, the result of a climbing mishap in the Sierras.

In his book, *You Gotta Keep Dancin'*, Tim answers a question many people have asked over and over, "Haven't You Been Healed?"

> "For years, people have asked me, 'Haven't you prayed to the Lord for healing?'
>
> "My obvious answer: 'Of course.'
>
> " 'Why do you think he hasn't healed you?' "
>
> " 'He has.' "
>
> " 'But I thought you were still in pain.' "
>
> " 'I am.'"
>
> " 'I don't understand.' "
>
> "I have prayed hundreds, if not thousands, of times for the Lord to heal me—and he finally healed me of the need to be healed." I had discovered a peace inside the pain.[29]

Tim's revelation of healing comes from a heart so surrendered to God's will that he no longer needs to be healed in the way *Tim* desires. His healing is now in line with God's healing. That is where I find myself after all these years of pain and suffering.

To quote my dear friend, Nancy Missler, "He has wounded me in my life, but only in order to heal me."

Look for miracles and answered prayer not only in the actual answer you requested, but in the perceived answer God knows is best for you.

Chapter 4
I Surrender All

I Surrender All

All to Jesus I surrender; All to him I freely give.
I will ever love and trust Him,
In His presence daily live.
I surrender all. I surrender all. All to Thee,
my blessed Saviour,
I surrender all.

Author, Judson W. Van de Venter, 1855-1939,
Composer, Winfield S. Weeden, 1847-1908

One surgery I went through on April 15, 2003, brought an entirely new concept of surrender to my understanding. My sternum, or the breast-bone holding the rib cage together, had been sawed in half to open my chest cavity for open-heart surgery. When the surgery is performed, the surgeon pulls the rib cage back together and "wires" it up so it can heal.

With all the complications of my first surgery, the sternum did not heal completely, but instead, healed in two pieces with merely cartilage holding it together. The movement of the bone was causing me additional chest pain, adding confusion to my symptoms. A heart surgeon, Dr. Nisco, who had assisted in my care had to go in, clean out the scar tissue, re-cut the bone, and put my sternum back together so it could heal properly. It had only been a year since my original double-bypass, open-heart surgery.

When my husband and I first met with Dr. Nisco and saw the results of the CT scan, we asked him if he saw this often—a sternum that did not heal together.

"No, this rarely happens." He turned to me as he shut off the light illuminating the x-ray film of my sternum. "You know, some people have one major thing go wrong with their health. Some may have a couple of major health issues. But with you, everything turns out to be a major health issue." His genuine concern was evidence of his soft tenure and sympathy as he handed me the consent form for surgery.

Many people have asked me if I was scared when facing yet another surgery, encountering possible death from a heart attack, or experiencing complications of multiple heart procedures being performed on me. My answer over time evolved, as with each setback, the feelings I experienced grew and developed into what I believe is the completion I felt as I faced this unexpected surgery.

Surrender, when totally understood, reveals another dimension of freedom. I was wheeled into the pre-op room with a total peace. I shared jokes along with my faith, and smiles along with my grimaces from pain. I can say I actually believe that I finally reached completion of my surrender. To be so out of control and so free from anxiety comes when you have surrendered everything. God now has one hundred percent of me and my life and my future. Once I gave it all to Him, I no longer feared what could happen to me. People tend to think that surrendering all is to give up all, but complete surrender brings enormous freedom.

I spoke with a friend a while back who was dealing with several heart-breaking trials. Her mom had been diagnosed with a fast-moving cancer; her niece, only days after being married, had to say goodbye to her new husband as he was deployed to Iraq; and another niece just had a baby girl who was born with Down syndrome. This friend called me after her birthday and shared how she retreated to her bedroom when her husband tried to surprise her with birthday festivities.

"I just didn't want to celebrate after all that was happening around me. I wanted to be alone, so I stayed in my bedroom and cried." She told me after always giving so much, she now reached a point where she could no longer give. Her only escape was to lock out everyone and take the time to cry and mourn. I truly believe that when we come to this point of brokenness, we must learn from our pain that all God wants is for us to *surrender*.

The word surrender is commonly understood as meaning giving up possession of something into the power of another, or to relinquish control completely. It's usually thought of in a cowardly or feeble context.

In an excerpt taken from Nancy Missler's book, *Private Worship, The Key to Joy*, Nancy describes why surrender is necessary to grow closer to God.

> Years ago, in one of David Wilkerson's newsletters, there was an article entitled, "The Making of a Man of God." I've never forgotten that intriguing title because, in a nutshell, this is what God is trying to do in all of our lives - make us men and women of God. If we really want to know how one becomes a "man of God," we have only to look at Jesus. This means that, at some point in our walk with the Lord, we too will experience rejection, confusion and loneliness just as Jesus did. Each of these situations will provide us with a greater opportunity to die a little more to our self and to grow a little more in grace and the image of God.
>
> John 12:24 validates this principle. Total surrender and relinquishment seem to be the cost of "becoming a man of God." Surrender Is Key: When God calls us

> to surrender all to Him, He is simply asking us to give back the life that He granted us in the first place. In other words, we're not being forced to lay our lives down; it's a choice that we are making out of our own free will and out of our love for Him.
>
> When all is said and done, I truly believe we will not only be judged by what we did for Him, but by how much we surrendered to Him, how much we loved Him and how much our hearts and lives were totally yielded to Him.[30]

A heart yielded to Him will exhibit a power we can draw only from the Lord. This power is a result of surrender and it is evident on the outside as well as the inside.

During one of my hospital stays for a heart catheterization, I had to actually go through two procedures over two days. The first catheterization revealed an unexpected blockage that had to be cleared out. Because it was performed at an outpatient facility adjacent to the hospital, my cardiologist could not do the repair. I had to be wheeled over to the hospital, admitted to a room, and the angioplasty needed to clear the blockage and stent it would have to be done the next day.

A heart catheterization requires a wire and catheter to be threaded through the femur artery in your upper thigh. If this artery were to start bleeding, you could quickly bleed to death. After any heart procedure, the patient needs to lie *completely flat* for a certain period of time. If there was no intervention, the time may only be one to three hours. But if anything has to be cleared out or stented, the time will be much longer.

In order to keep the original tubing in my leg and prevent bleeding, I had to lie flat in a hospital room before the procedure that next day. Between the first day and then after the blockage was cleared, the total time I remained flat was 36 hours! No moving my right leg where the catheter was placed, no picking up my head, no sitting up, and no activity that could cause the femur artery to bleed. It had to heal.

My son Jonathan spoke with me by phone. He was only 15 at the time, but he had well-seasoned wisdom. "Mom, concentrate on your left leg," he told me over the phone.

What do you mean, Jonathan?" I was perplexed.

"Well, you can't move your right leg, but you can move your left leg a little so just think about your left leg and move it as often as you can." I tried his suggestion and it helped to pass the hours.

My 36 hours ended right at 11:00 p.m. that next night. I was slowly allowed to sit up to be sure I didn't pass out. The freedom was refreshing and I walked the halls just to get myself moving again.

The very next morning, an aide came into my room. Betty was a shy, soft-natured woman who stopped by to speak with me often. She was a new Christian and liked to talk about her faith. I was sitting in front of the window trying to absorb some of the sunshine shining in and wondering what it would be like to smell fresh air.

"You look so peaceful sitting there with your brown, curly hair shining in the sunlight. It's almost like I am looking at Jesus," she commented. "I wish I had what you have." She knew what I had just been through and yet was amazed at how happy and content I appeared.

"You do have what I have," I offered her. "You are a Christian who has asked Jesus to inhabit your heart and life. He gives all of us the same portion of faith, peace, and trust. We all have free access to His strength but it takes surrender of our will and desire to fight to let Him take over and handle all that we struggle with."

Betty stayed a bit and talked with me. I so wanted her to know that surrender is such a powerful opposite to what the world knows surrender to be.

Kenneth W. Osbeck, in his book *Amazing Grace, 366 Inspiring Hymn Stories for Daily Devotions*, writes this about surrender based on the hymn, "I Surrender All:"

> The Bible teaches us that brokenness is a prerequisite to blessing and usefulness. No one ever achieves spiritual greatness until he has fully surrendered himself to God. Victorious living comes only as we abandon ourselves to the Lordship of Christ, becoming His loving bond slave. God's best for our lives is not the result of struggle. Rather, it is simply the acceptance of His perfect will and the recognition of His authority in every area of our lives.[31]

Victorious living is the result of painfully enduring a full surrendering of your self to God. You may look at people you know are suffering in many ways, even your own suffering, and ask, "Where is this victorious living? I have suffered much pain and gone through many trials and still I cannot see any hope of victory. When will it come?" It will come once you recognize what hinders peace and how to give all the offending problems to the Lord.

When I was a couple of years into my illness, I felt I needed to talk to a Christian counselor—someone who was neutral and could help clear the way for my thoughts to be freed from some of the terrors that caused me to stumbled. I found one and set up the first few appointments. One assignment he gave me that was supposed to last a week lasted only a half day after I saw through its purpose.

He had instructed me to keep a sheet of paper for the week with two columns on it. One side would be a list of all the times I got depressed, angry, nervous, anxious, or mad. The other side would show whatever situation caused me the emotion. After writing down a few incidents, I understood his purpose—each situation that caused me grief was something I could not change. Each was a difficult issue that could not be avoided. There was nothing I could do. I had to let God take care of the things that rattled me and the way to do this was to surrender my trust, my life, my abilities, my entire being to God only.

Judson Van De Venter, author of "I Surrender All," wrote the following after surrendering his many talents to the Lord:

> For some time, I had struggled between developing my talents in the field of art and going into full-time evangelistic work. At last the pivotal hour of my life came, and I surrendered all. A new day was ushered into my life, I became an evangelist and discovered down deep in my soul a talent hitherto unknown to me. God had hidden a song in my heart, and touching a tender chord, He caused me to sing.[32]

When God knows you have finally surrendered all, you will also know because the victory that is meant for you will bring the freedom of complete joy.

As I hugged the shaken body of a grievous mom shattered by the weight of a multitude of sorrows, I felt her despair. "I am trying so hard to be strong for my kids," she sobbed. How desperately I wanted to convince her that she did not have to be strong. That she did not have to strive so painfully to battle the war raging all around her.

"You don't have to be strong. Just surrender and let God be your strength. He can do it but we can't. We don't have to." I whispered the words in her ear hoping to feel her tense, weighted shoulders ease into retreat, letting God bear the turmoil. But she couldn't let go and I held onto her a little while more, desperate to share the peace of God with her.

I reflected on the past few years of illness and tried to figure out how it was that I obtained this peace. It is a peace that has freed me from trying to rely on my own strength. As I played back all the episodes of trials and tests dealt to me while I dodged heart attacks time and time again, I failed to find one specific event that pushed me through the door of surrender. I could see that it took day after day of physical pain and emotional agony to transform me into an empty vessel with only God left to save me.

I had no idea what God was doing in my life. I could not see the end of the goal. I knew nothing of God's purpose. All I had to do was let go and let God take me to the place He had for me.

I dislike roller coasters and vow never to ride one again. But the times I did, the terrible fear of being at the top and not knowing where I would end up, or how tumultuous it would be getting there, made me shake with fear. The first time I rode one, the blood seemed to drain from my very soul. With my hands gripping the sides of the car, I screamed all the way down only to find out all was well as the cars slowed to stop. It was like being in a free fall and wondering if the cord would hold me back from certain death.

So now I choose not to ride a roller coaster. Nor would I try my luck at bungee jumping, hang gliding, or any other death-defying activity. But the way my life has changed since first getting sick is like riding that roller coaster—only not by choice. What can I do? I'm at the top and the car must go down for the ride to continue and ultimately come to an end. Each trial I face is so different, it's like a whole new ride with more unknown twists and turns. There's no going back once the car is put into motion.

Life is just that way. We are put into motion the day we are born. The ride will encounter sudden turns, hills to climb, unknown plunges over steep slopes, and surprises at every corner. How can anyone keep themselves in a state of peace and composure while the ride continues? How can a person hold on when, for them, the next pitfall signifies imminent failure or destruction?

I became so wanting my illness to end or at least "begin" to end that I prayed for God to take it away. My desperation sent me to an answer from the Lord that I had heard before. His answers always pointed the way back to Him—back to surrender.

One Sunday morning in May of 2003, God spoke to me in a quiet, calm voice and directed me to read Jeremiah 14:19-22. The words in brackets are what He instructed me to replace so I could make these verses a very personal message:

> Have You completely rejected Judah [me]? Or have You loathed Zion [me]? Why have You stricken us [me] so that we are [I am] beyond healing? We [I] waited for peace, but nothing good came; And for a time of healing, but behold, terror! We [I] know our [my] wickedness, O LORD, The iniquity of our fathers, for we [I] have sinned against You. Do not despise us, [me] for Your own name's sake; Do not disgrace the throne of Your glory; Remember and do not annul Your covenant with us. [me] Are there any among the idols of the nations who give rain? Or can the heavens grant showers? Is it not You, O LORD our [my] God? Therefore we [I] hope in You, For You are the one who has done all these things (NASB).

This was some great praying on Jeremiah's part. Much like his kindred brother Job, Jeremiah acknowledges that only God can control much of the essentials in life. Only God can facilitate what happens each day we wake and live and work and play.

In her book *Out of Control and Loving it!*, Lisa Bevere talks about how God often "shakes us to wake us."

> When God shakes us to wake us, we often find ourselves surrounded by the unfamiliar and unfriendly. God wakes us up from the secure by pushing us out of our comfort zone. By comfort zone I am referring to all that is familiar, expected, constant and under our own control.
>
> We are comfortable when what we expect happens. We enjoy being understood and supported by those around us. We prefer to have a constant source of financial provision.
>
> When God's flight training began in earnest in my life, I felt as if there was nothing to hold on to. It seemed my life was a sea of uncertainty. Everything that had been constant was in upheaval or transition. Our finances were lacking. Socially we were shunned. I felt alone, isolated, misunderstood and persecuted. I prayed and cried out to the Lord for direction, only to hear my unanswered questions echoing back at me, I could find no rest. I was uncomfortable because I was experiencing God's shaking in every aspect of my life. His shaking removes what is temporary and leaves only what is of His kingdom. When God has shaken an area in your life, don't try to rebuild it yourself. Allow Him to restore only those things He wants to establish in your life.[33]

Being out of control *is* being surrendered. But as Lisa Bevere notes, God wants us to let Him restore and rebuild what we may lose in our relinquishing. And when we feel we have given more than our share or have surrendered all that we can, there may still be some small part of our life we try to hold onto. We want to at least have something left in our control, some area that we feel God cannot shake or amputate. Yet, to be totally out of control, to have nothing left, is truly a point where you can realize all that you have is in God's power.

"You can't say Jesus is all you need until Jesus is all you've got," said Mother Theresa. This amazing woman truly knew the reality of needing only God to live life. In her years of dedication to helping the dying and impoverished people of India, she understood the value of relying on God and Him alone.

Imagine the powerful effect we can have if we suffer enormous tragedy not only once or twice, but also through relentless, chronic suffering on a daily basis. If we choose bitterness, anger, and depression, our suffering is rendered powerless and inconsequential.

Yet, if we choose to abdicate all our strife to God alone, and arise from the trials with joy and laughter, people around us will want to know "How? How do you keep so upbeat in the face of tragedy?" We can then give an answer and point to total dependence upon our God. Who benefits? We, ourselves, through strengthening our faith and those on whom we impress the power of prayer and surrender.

Sometimes surrender can bring us a more worthy gift than we can conceive. My letter carrier was a sweet, dear lady who even wrote me a note asking forgiveness when she inadvertently delivered someone else's mail to my house. I can hardly think of anyone as kind as her.

But one day, her life began a shaking process that would turn everything upside down. Within one month, her husband announced he wanted a divorce, her only son, a successful financial advisor—was sent to prison for embezzlement, and she was diagnosed with amyotrophic lateral sclerosis, or ALS also known as Lou Gehrig's disease named after the famed baseball player whose struggle with this disease and death in 1941 brought it to national attention. ALS is an incurable, progressive degenerative neurological disorder. For reasons that are not understood, the nerve cells of the brain and spinal cord that control voluntary muscle movement gradually deteriorate. As a result, muscles waste away, leading to paralysis and death, usually in two to five years.[34]

I can't think of how much worse things could get for her. Still, in her suffering, she was so out of control and surrendered to God. She was not concerned about herself but of others as shown by this letter she sent me:

Dear Cindy,

I have asked God to bless me with the right words to express what I need to say. Perhaps you have heard that I have been diagnosed with Lou Gehrig's disease. I plan on taking different steps to fight the progression of this disease. However, the medical doctors don't give me any hope. You may already know that ALS is a disease that affects the nerves in your spinal cord, which sends pulses to your muscles. Eventually these neurons die and your muscles become more and more weak as time goes on. Anyway, to live in reality, should my efforts to stop the progression not work and God prefers to take me home to Him soon; I say soon because the doctors say two to five years, I would like you to know I believe it would please God, if I am a compatible match with you . . . I would like to do all of the tests and fill out the paperwork to make sure you get the use of my heart. I don't mean to give you any false hope. I do hope you will pray on this.

Love, your sister in Christ,
Shelia

Shelia wrote this letter on March 15, 2005. I can't properly express how her words made me feel. Here I was, complaining about my suffering, whining about being out of control. And here she is, willing to give me *her heart*.

I committed to pray for her to be healed. How could I even imagine her life for mine? I so wanted God to give back what she offered—complete surrender. I wanted her to be rewarded for her selflessness.

On September 25, 2005, six months later, I received an email from one of Shelia's co-workers.

> Hello all,
>
> Remember Shelia that was diagnosed from 2 specialists that she had Lou Gehrig's disease and she had to quit work, and was not able to walk very good? Well, good news. Another Doctor re-tested her for Lymes Disease (symptoms are both quite the same) and she has that, in fact Acute Lyme Disease. She will start antibiotic treatments and should be doing much, much better in a year or less. She had been tested 4 months ago for it, but the lab did not catch it. This last test was with a lab in California that specializes in Lymes disease. So does that make your day or what!!!!! I am doing the Happy Dance (not a pretty site but I just can't help it)
>
> Becky

Shelia gave up her heart and God gave it back to her with more love than it could ever hold before. These are the times the painful events in our lives allow us to see God's hand and power. "You have turned for me my mourning into dancing" (Psalm 30: 11 NASB). Sometimes we dance with broken bones as David spoke of in Psalm 51:8: "Let the bones dance which thou hast broken."

David, although a "man after God's own heart," knew the pain of brokenness.

David Swartz, in his book, *Dancing With Broken Bones*, describes King David's dilemma as not just a spiritual or physical brokenness, but an opportunity for God to prove His love and care for us:

> For all of us, spiritual growth sometimes means going down a path we would much rather detour around. It means being broken into unstable pieces. But brokenness need not always hit with one great big blow like as it did here in David's life. In fact, if we look closely, we will see incidents and relationships scattered across his life that should have reminded him regularly of his deep dependence on God. His spiritual bones were broken gradually.
>
> But although David learned the hard way, he did learn. Christians everywhere sustain the same kinds of losses—*but* there is good news! No matter how broken we become, God can put all the pieces back together again. He alone can make us whole.[35]

A broken heart, a broken life, a broken relationship, and a broken promise—all these things can lead to a loss of hope. And when your life breaks apart in front of you, the last thing you want to do is let go. Most of us would want to do whatever it takes to fix it. And although we do need to live and do whatever we can, the root of our success is in our ability to lose control. Dependence on God is a good thing—not a weakness. Being broken is a pathway to growth—not defeat!

Years ago, I was driving through New York City. Stuck in traffic, I looked out onto the sidewalk, and slumped up against the cold, brick wall, was the figure of a man lying on the cruel, gray, cement sidewalk. An empty wine bottle was clenched under his arm—testifying of his empty life. People walked over him, occasionally kicking his legs out of their way.

Was he alive? I wondered. I couldn't tell if he was breathing.

My car lunged forward as I grabbed a chance to move on. The dark figure weighed on my thoughts. I can still picture him even now—a child of God, a living human being.

One moment in time and one small space in this huge city, painted the very core of bitterness and anger that seeped from every crevice. The intensity of its sharp taste burned as I reflected on what our world has become. I mulled over the distressing statements often heard from people struggling to get through their tattered lives:

"No one will ever tell me what to do."

"I run my own life. Where is God when you need him?"

"I can't even pray anymore—what's the use? Even the sight of a church turns me away."

"What type of a God would leave me here to suffer? Nothing will change. Nothing will ever get better. When I get to hell, I'll be ready. I've had lots of practice here."

The voices echo. People's pain covers the surface of their wounds like tightly bound gauze, oozing with burdens too difficult to bear. Bitterness has taken root. Can we as Christians become trapped by the same bitterness? Are we not susceptible to the anger that feeds its roots?

Many instances can be attributed to the root of bitterness—personal losses such as financial problems, housing, death of a family member or spouse, infertility, loss of employment, no transportation, poor health, and a loss of sense of home—having to relocate. Then there are emotional losses. A friendship ends painfully, marital problems lead to divorce, children grow rebellious, and family members betray us.

The root of anger and bitterness often stems from—and feeds off of—some kind of loss. Even as we strive to develop our relationship with the Lord, we can experience spiritual loss, which can be the most forbidding loss leading to bitterness.

> "See to it that no one comes short of the grace of God; that no root of bitterness springing up causes trouble, and by it many be defiled;" (Hebrews 12:15 NASB)

So how do we destroy bitterness—root and all?

In the book of Job, chapters 38–42, Job describes God's great works. When we look at what the Lord can do compared to our abilities, we see that only He can reach far enough to destroy the roots of bitterness so deeply embedded in our lives.

> Have you ever in your life commanded the morning, and caused the dawn to know its place? Have you entered into the springs of the sea, or walked in the recesses of the deep? Have you entered the storehouses of the snow, or have you seen the storehouses of the hail? Can you bind the chains of the Pleiades, or loose the cords of Orion? Can you lead forth a constellation in its season, and guide the Bear with her satellites? Can you lift up your voice to the clouds, so that an abundance of water will cover you? Can you send forth lightnings that they may go and say to you, "Here we are"? (NASB)

When I meet with people who are dismayed about their lives and the pain each day delivers, I try to share how my complete surrender sustains me because of God's power. Often, their response is that they aren't like me and cannot give control to God as I had. They express defeat at what they feel is an impossible task.

Besides what I have to offer through my testimony, which continuously builds on surmounting trials, I share with them Paul's recollection of Abraham's faith when he stood on the promises of God:

> For what does the Scripture say? ABRAHAM BELIEVED GOD, AND IT WAS CREDITED TO HIM AS RIGHTEOUSNESS. Without becoming weak in faith he contemplated his own body, now as good as dead since he was about a hundred years old, and the deadness of Sarah's womb; yet, with respect to the promise of God, he did not waver in unbelief but grew strong in faith, giving glory to God, and being fully assured that what God had promised, He was able also to perform. Therefore IT WAS ALSO CREDITED TO HIM AS RIGHTEOUSNESS (Romans 4:3,18-22 NASB).

Nancy Missler wrote an insightful article about surrender:

> Abandonment to God's will means a kind of weightless floating, having released all of our personal clutching for emotional and intellectual security, all of our personal needs to know and understand, all of our personal disturbances about being right, all of our personal humiliations at being wrong, making mistakes and looking stupid, and all of our personal frustrations over being denied what we thought God promised. It's being completely dead to all of our own "self" interests, passions, prejudices, pleasures and reputation and choosing, instead, to leave everything in God's hand.

> Fenelon, the great sixteenth-century author and saint, expresses it this way: "Inward peace comes [only] with absolute surrender to the will of God. ...*The reason you feel so agitated is that you do not accept everything that happens to you with complete trust in God.* Put everything in His hand, and offer yourself to Him as a sacrifice. ...Until you reach a point of surrender, your life will be full of trouble and aggravation. ...So give your heart wholly to God and you will find peace and joy in the Holy Spirit." (*The Seeking Heart*, Fenelon)[36]

Many choices come our way each day as we battle through life. Often the walls of despair become too high too see over.

When my son was little, we loved to visit the local corn maze in the fall. Crisp air, robust apples, carved pumpkins lighting the way, and endless corn stalks lined the opening to a corn maze acres deep.

Without a map, children and parents were instructed where to start and where to exit the maze. "No breaking through the outside walls," the guide informed us.

Jonathan ran off with his friends and before I even had a sense of direction, he had gone through and exited the maze three times.

Trailing all the others, a friend and I became equally frustrated at the twisting turns and unfamiliar pathways. Finally, worn out and disenchanted by the fun of it, I broke through an outside wall, letting both of us out. I propped up as much of the corn as I could to cover up my folly.

Sometimes we can only look up past the high towering walls and plead with God to guide us through to the end. Breaking through a clouded wall of life's frustrations will not bring victory.

Since my illness, I have gained a new understanding of surrender. I have learned that surrendering all is something we have to determine to do every day. Knowing that my life hangs loosely here on earth, I have learned to surrender my husband, my son, my family and friends, my goals and desires, and my very life.

Yet when I think I have truly given all my ambitions over to God, another tragedy strikes and I find I've taken back some of what I surrendered. Unlike sacrifice, which puts the attention on our efforts to please God, obedience hurts. Obedience requires us to tear off pieces of ourselves as we surrender all to the Lord. In Deuteronomy 4:4, the Lord promises to keep safe those who cleave to Him: "But all of you who held fast to the LORD your God are still alive today" (NIV).

Think of how many new beginnings God gives us each time we surrender something we have held onto so tightly. *Letting go* is *taking back* the life God wants us to live.

5 Chapter 5
One is *Not* the Loneliest Number

One

'Cause one is the loneliest number that you'll ever do
One is the loneliest number, worse than two
One is the loneliest, number one is the loneliest
Number one is the loneliest number that you'll ever do

Three Dog Night, "One" Three Dog Night, MCA Records,1969

I remember hearing this popular '60s song from Three Dog Night at the end of a week when I could have easily said, "Yes, one is the loneliest number." Sitting in the hospital for the umpteenth time, staring at the pallid green walls, I remembered how a friend who also endured a heart transplant described the confinement. I asked her how she was doing after five long weeks of being isolated in her hospital room.

"You mean my box?" she replied.

Her description caused me to look about my room as the walls seemed to close in on me.

How I wished they were any other color besides sea-foam green. How I wished I wasn't so lonely and isolated. Depression slithered about, wrapping itself around each corner.

Loneliness is a word with far more meaning than we realize. Being lonely conjures up thoughts of one person, alone in a room, forgotten by everyone. But loneliness is often much more. At times, the feeling of being so isolated and separated from friends, family, the outside world, and sometimes even God, drives us to an ultimate void. We can choose to drift deeper or we can choose to allow God's presence to saturate our days. I have been at this crossroad many times and sense I will visit this dilemma again and again.

During the hardest times of my battle with heart disease, I had lonely days in which I dragged my body from bed, weary at the thought of another day. I was tired and heavy with despair. My thoughts were of defeat and uselessness, wondering why I was even alive anymore. Many days I had a bottomless feeling that I was forgotten. Sometimes long periods went by where no one called, no one came by to visit, no one came to rescue me from the mundane routine of being home and alone. It wasn't as though people didn't care to minister to me, but everyone had families, and lives, and schedules. Being chronically ill or chronically anything gets old.

Being so alone, feeling so isolated and separated from friends and the outside world, I began to feel my joy slipping away. Larry Crabb, in his book *Shattered Dreams,* talks of the despondency pain and trials can bring;

> Nothing makes me feel more alone than personal pain. When I'm in the middle of shattered dreams, I often hear myself saying, "If you knew the anguish I feel, if you knew how desperate I am despite how together I look, you would not taunt me with the promise of joy. You would come to me in my pain and just be with me, saying by your silent presence that my pain is justified and so too is my loss of hope. An invitation to dream higher dreams is as cruel as talking to a pilgrim lost in the burning desert about water that does not exist."[37]

One day, self-pity began to boil over until I had no room for any other thoughts. I wasn't reading my Bible or praying, and I eventually spiraled into a depression fringing on the side of anger. I didn't even want anyone to look at me. This is the flavor of depression. Being so consumed with my own internal battles and external trials, I gave way to a pessimistic sense of inadequacy and total despondence. How does anyone return to the top of the hole dug by such a destructive state? I had only one choice left—use the solitude and lack of distractions to actually hear God—and God alone.

When I finally reached the end of all I had aspired to do, and when even my own voice was silenced, all distractions were gone and God's voice became intimate and close. Although alone, I could feel His presence wrapped around my feeble body.

Yes, there are medicines for depression, and chronic illness or emotional stresses may push a person's physiological state into a deficiency of certain chemicals in the brain. Medicines are sometimes needed. But the emotional and spiritual toll comes when we let go of the personal will to fight physically and the personal surrender to let God take control.

These feelings tend to be temporal examples and pose no real threat to a person's life. But depression can set in from loneliness and when it does, there is usually more than one cause.

Depression can come when deeper yearnings inside each person cry out for fulfillment. We desire friendship, companionship, comradeship—other people to share our experiences. There is also a tendency to seek a kinship in suffering—a "misery loves company" association. We want someone to understand our void and offer us some compassion or endowment that will replace our loneliness.

Many times during the years of hospital stays, doctor visits, lab appointments, a myriad of tests, and other appointments, I dreaded the shawl of loneliness that hung over my shoulders.

Many friends, family, and my faithful husband were there for me countless times. Gifts, cards, dinners, financial help, and other acts of kindness were lavished on me. Sometimes a friend would drive me to an appointment and stay with me until I was done. Physically I was not alone. But often I was emotionally lost into solitary suffering. "God, does anyone else have to go through this? When will it stop? When God?"

Questions of despair clouded my thoughts and prevented me from seeing that I was not really alone. God was—and is—always there for me. He is certainly bigger than the looming loneliness, keeping watch. He stays by my side and only wishes I would listen more to His communications.

Many people desperately want to hear God speaking. Our minds conjure up ideas of audible messages or direct dialogue with God. We wonder how God speaks."What language does He use?"

Oswald Chambers in his book, *My Utmost for His Highest*, has a focused description of how God speaks to us.

> There is no escape when our Lord speaks. He always comes using His authority and taking hold of our understanding. Has the voice of God come to you directly? If it has, you cannot mistake the intimate insistence with which it has spoken to you. God speaks in the language you know best— not through your ears, but through your circumstances.[38]

"Through our circumstances . . ." is a large ensemble of events, situations, and possibilities. I found many ways God spoke to me through my turmoil and pain once I was willing to "see" the more intricate ways He communicates.

C.S. Lewis, author and scholar, agrees:

> God whispers to us in our pleasures, speaks in our conscience, but shouts in our pains: it is His megaphone to rouse a deaf world.

In what other specific ways does a God who is infinite in wisdom, omnipresent, and creator of all things speak to us?

Through His Word:

Sitting in church before the service one Sunday morning, I pondered yet another heart procedure that was scheduled for the next day. Testing showed a massive blockage in the main artery of my heart. In a quiet whisper, I was led to open my Bible to Jeremiah 33:6. *Oh, what now, Lord, another inspirational verse?* I was cynical and unreceptive. But I read:

> Behold, I will bring it [you] health and cure, and I will cure them, [you] and will reveal unto them [you] the abundance of peace and truth. (Brackets are what the Lord told me to substitute to make it personal.)

That next day the procedure was done—but no blockage was found. God healed me just as He spoke to me through His Word.

Through God Speaking to Us in Our Minds

In December of 2001, only three months after first developing heart disease, I was praying for God to heal me. His reply, which I heard in my mind, was less then encouraging. "*I cannot heal you until you are ready to accept how I choose to heal you—and I am not finished yet!*"

Okay, I thought, I *will wait for You to be finished*. How pompous I must have sounded to the Lord. Instead of a sweet smelling aroma rising to Him in the heavens, I was like a noisome complainer! What I could not comprehend was that His promise of healing would not take on *my* design and resolution, but *His* will and desire. His timing and His ways often do not make any sense to our minds. What seemed to be an answer with an ending, "I am not finished yet," was actually an admonition for me to continue listening to Him and finding my source of endurance only through him.

Though I did not then realize the power of His words, I know now that His promise has been fulfilled over and over, and I take comfort in His care.

Through God's Creation in Nature

The day I came home from the hospital in the summer of 2005, after having died and been brought back twice, I sat on a chair in my backyard. The warmth of the sun soothed me and I prayed quietly, asking the Lord if He would allow me to live much longer.

Suddenly I heard the call of a hawk and looked up to the sky. Three hawks were circling above me—not a common sight in my suburban neighborhood. I thought of the Trinity and took solace. "You will fly free like the hawks above," the Lord seemed to speak to me.

A week later, I stepped out my front door and found a very long hawk feather from a very large hawk. What are the odds of one of those hawks just happening to lose a feather in just the right spot, with just the right wind to cause it to land on my front porch?

Another week later, on the way home from church, three hawks swooped down over our van as my husband drove home. They almost crashed into our windshield. Again the Lord whispered to me, *You will fly free like the hawks above*. A few weeks later I received a miracle heart transplant! If I had not received that heart transplant, I would have surely died.

Through Physical Items

On one particularly tough day I sat despondent, staring out the window. I watched as the letter carrier delivered the mail to our mailbox. "Go out and get the mail," I was prompted by the Lord—a task not done easily for me. I was so bad off that walking to the mailbox was almost impossible. But I trudged down the steps and got the mail.

By the time I got back to the house, I was so short of breath I collapsed on the couch. In the pile were two greeting cards—one from a dear friend, the other from an anonymous sender. Both were postmarked the same day, from different states, and in different colored envelopes. But they were the exact same card! What was the verse on the front?

> I will lift up my eyes to the mountains; from where shall my help come? My help comes from the LORD, who made heaven and earth. (Psalm 121:1-2 NIV)

That verse was exactly what I needed to hear. Receiving those two cards on the same day was like receiving a personal letter from God!

Through God's Chastening

Coming home from a doctor's appointment one day, sobbing uncontrollably, I begged the Lord to speak to me and tell me what to do. The doctor I had at the time, and many previous ones I had seen for my heart condition, were all so callous and intent on blaming my symptoms on psychiatric problems. The Lord instantly put an idea in my head to call a girlfriend. *Why, Lord? She doesn't know anything about heart disease!*

Stubbornly, I opposed the Lord's prompting until I finally called her. She had a friend whose husband is a cardiologist and a Christian! The end result was finding the doctor I still see today. He is not only is a gem, but has saved my life countless times.

Through Uncertainty

Waiting one evening at the hospital to have an emergency heart procedure, I became frustrated as one emergency after another came and went and my own procedure was delayed several times. After seven hours of waiting, I finally asked the Lord to allow His will and give me a peace about the outcome. *Should I go through with this, Lord?*

Soon after I prayed, a nurse came into my room and informed me the procedure had to be cancelled. Instead of being angry, I was relieved. That next day the doctors figured out something else was wrong and the problem was easily treated with medication.

When we feel the most alone and even distant from God, He is still there, just as close as He always was and is. When we feel like there is nothing left to our very existence, God's presence can saturate our days. Truly being void of all our support systems opens up the entrance for the power of God's infinite presence. Whatever your trial, no matter what burden suppresses your desire to go on living, you truly are not alone.

When those memorable lines from Three Dog Night chimed from the radio, I knew it wasn't true. I knew that even as God exists, there is never a time that any person on this vast earth is ever really alone.

Another unforgettable song exemplifies the way God speaks to our inner soul during times of distress. Written by Elizabeth P.

Prentiss, "More Love to Thee" is a hymn inspired by a lifetime of great suffering.

> Mrs. Elizabeth Payson Prentiss, born in Portland, Maine, on October 26, 1818, was known throughout her life as a saintly woman, who continually practiced the presence of Christ. Those who knew her best described her as "a very, bright-eyed, little woman, with a keen sense of humor, who cared more to shine in her own happy household than in a wide circle of society." Though Elizabeth was strong in spirit, she was frail in body. Throughout her life she was a near invalid, scarcely knowing a moment free of pain. She once wrote these words:
>
> "I see now that to live for God, whether one is allowed ability to be actively useful or not, is a great thing, and that it is a wonderful mercy to be allowed even to suffer, if thereby one can glorify Him."
>
> "More Love to Thee" was written during a time of great personal sorrow. While ministering to a church in New York City during the 1850s, the Prentis' lost a child, and then a short time later their youngest child also died. For weeks, Elizabeth was inconsolable, and in her diary she wrote, "Empty hands, a worn-out, exhausted body, and unutterable longings to flee from a world that has so many sharp experiences."
>
> During this period of grief, Mrs. Prentiss began meditating upon the story of Jacob in the Old Testament, and how God met him in a very special way during his moments of sorrow and deepest need. She prayed earnestly that she too might have a similar experience.[39]

Her prayer for this personal knowledge inspired a poem. It was first printed as a leaflet in 1869 and later published in the hymnal *Songs of Devotion*. "More Love to Thee" is translated in many languages and still touches many with the message of sorrow and love.

More Love to Thee

More l*ove to Thee, O Christ, More love to Thee!*
Hear Thou the prayer I make on bended knee.
This is my earnest plea: More love, O Christ, to Thee;
More love to Thee, More love to Thee!

Once earthly joy I craved, Sought peace and rest;
Now Thee alone I seek; Give what is best.
This all my prayer shall be: More love,
O Christ to Thee;
More love to Thee, More love to Thee!

Let sorrow do its work, come grief or pain;
Sweet are Thy messengers, sweet their refrain,
When they can sing with me: More love,
O Christ, to Thee;
More love to Thee, More love to Thee!

I believe when we read prose such as this and we experience isolation caused by any kind of circumstance in our lives, we can choose to follow and love God just as Mrs. Prentiss did. Not only do *we* love God, but also resting in *His* love removes the fears that come with painful times.

The reason it's so important to know God's Love
is because when we see His handprint of Love in every

> aspect of our lives, we'll never fear what He might allow into our lives. Nancy Missler[40]

How can we possibly *tune into* these ways God speaks to us once we realize *how* He speaks?

One such story of revelation is found in the Old Testament book of Genesis. The story of an Egyptian slave, Hagar and her unhappy plight, ultimately led to an encounter with an angel of God that marked a theological commencement for the people of her day.

"Hagar" means fugitive, immigrant, or stranger, and that she was as her life as an Egyptian woman turned to a life of slavery. Hagar was cut off from her home and identity as she was forced to become Sarah's handmaid (Abraham's wife).

Hagar was considered a concubine—a woman who co-habits with a man or functions as a second wife without the legal standing of a full wife. Sarah gave Hagar to Abraham to acquire a child through her for herself (Genesis 16:2).

Sarah made life hard for Hagar. She wanted to bear Abraham a child and as she grew older and older, she became desperate. Although Sarah gave Hagar to Abraham to bear a child for them both, she held contempt for the woman who would fulfill her husband's desire.

Genesis 16:6-10,14, gives a detailed account of Hagar's angelic visitation:

> So Sarai treated her harshly, and she fled from her presence. Now the angel of the LORD found her by a spring of water in the wilderness, by the spring on the way to Shur. He said, "Hagar, Sarai's maid, where have you come from and where are you going?" And she said, "I am fleeing from the presence of my mistress

> Sarai." Then the angel of the LORD said to her, "Return to your mistress, and submit yourself to her authority." Moreover, the angel of the LORD said to her, "I will greatly multiply your descendants so that they will be too many to count." Then she called the name of the LORD who spoke to her, "You are a God who sees," for she said, "Have I even remained alive here after seeing Him?" Therefore the well was called Beer-lahai-roi; behold, it is between Kadesh and Bered." (NASB)

Hagar recognized that a deity had spoken to her. She then called God, "El Roi, You are the God who sees me," and she named the well where she met God "Beer Lahi Roi," or "well of the Living One Who sees me."

In her book, *Lost Women of the Bible*, Carolyn Custis James discusses this time in Hagar's life where loneliness was overcome by her new, intimate relationship to God.

> In her encounter with the Angel of God, Hagar received dignity and meaning. The simple but unchanging truth that God's eyes were fixed on her empowered her with a kind of freedom no one could ever take away. She was not alone. She *did* matter.
>
> No one else in Scripture—male or female—ever names God. Hagar does. The new name she gives to God expresses her most basic theological conviction: she is not invisible to God.[41]

Hagar was an Egyptian slave woman—yet God met her where she was. He called her by her name. She had no previous knowledge of God, she was pregnant with a "rebel" child, and she was a woman. We think God cannot speak to us if we are turned away from Him, or not living up to certain standards as a

Christian or are living in some kind of sin or rebellion. What do you feel keeps God from speaking to you? He is always speaking to you. You just have to listen!

Carolyn Custis James finishes her story about Hagar with this sagely advice:

> It just goes to show how lonely life can be amid the hustle and bustle of activities, errands, crowds, and friendships. Even inside a good marriage or close friendship, there's still a dimension of isolation we cannot escape. For all of us, there are plenty of wilderness experiences when we suffer symptoms of isolation and insignificance. For all of us, there are inevitable moments when, even surrounded by loving family and friends, we feel invisible or go through something alone. A surgery, divorce, a death, a failure. Those sleepless nights, those closet moments, those tears we shed in private. What we wouldn't give to find Hagar's spring and to be found by the Angel of the Lord.[42]

Sometimes it is in the hardest times in life that God lets us know He is a God who sees us.

How much did I still have to suffer through? Questions like that place my eyes on my situation. We can get so caught up in our pain and suffering that we can't hear God speaking to us. Like Nancy's statement: "The reason it's so important to know God's Love is because when we see His handprint of Love in every aspect of our lives, we'll never fear what He might allow into our lives." We have to realize God loves us and whatever is happening He is a God who sees us! And He speaks to us in so many ways.

Larry Crabb stresses the ability to see past our shattered dreams, pain and loneliness:

> The dream to experience God rises from deep within me. I see the possibility of living beyond shattered dreams.[43]

Lonely? Love God. Let Him in so He can dissipate the loneliness crippling you. One is *not* the loneliest number!

Chapter 6
"Ya Gotta' Laugh"

Why a chapter about laughing? Since 2001, my life no longer rests in the category of "normal." Trials I hoped would not happen until I had already lived many long years of happiness, health, and vibrancy, have now propelled me into the future. Brittle bones, memory loss, swollen feet and legs, fatigue, and many other symptoms constantly plague me. These maladies make me try even harder to find ways to combat the assault.

Laughter is just one of my defenses.

Laughter, according to the American Heritage Dictionary, means, "To express certain emotions, especially mirth or delight; to show or feel amusement or good humor; to feel a triumphant or exultant sense of well-being. The Merriam-Webster's Dictionary also describes laughter as "An expression of merriment," or as "To be of a kind that inspires joy."

And the word "silly" (of which I think of myself) in the Greek is *selig*, which means blessed, happy, or blissful.

My hope is to make you laugh and to inspire you with joy—"the joy of the LORD." Remember one of my anchor verses: "The joy of the LORD is your strength" (Nehemiah 8:10b NASB).

Laughter is also good medicine.

What Happens When We Laugh? We change physiologically when we laugh. We stretch muscles throughout our face and body, our pulse and blood pressure go up, and we breathe faster, sending more oxygen to our tissues. And laughter appears to burn calories, too. Maciej Buchowski, a researcher from Vanderbilt University, conducted a small study in which he measured the amount of calories expended in laughing. It turned out that 10-15 minutes of laughter burned 50 calories.[44]

Health benefits of humor and laughter: "Laughter activates the chemistry of the will to live and increases our capacity to fight disease. Laughing relaxes the body and reduces problems associated with high blood pressure, strokes, arthritis, and ulcers. Some research suggests that laughter may also reduce the risk of heart disease. Historically, research has shown that distressing emotions (depression, anger, anxiety, and stress) are all related to heart disease. A study done at the University of Maryland Medical Center suggests that a good sense of humor and the ability to laugh at stressful situations helps mitigate the damaging physical effects of distressing emotions."

A good hearty laugh can help: reduce stress, lower blood pressure, elevate mood, boost immune system, improve brain functioning, protect the heart, connect you to others, foster instant relaxation, make you feel good. Laughter decreases stress hormones and increases infection-fighting antibodies. It increases our attentiveness, heart rate, and pulse.[45]

Why wouldn't you want to have a good laugh? Here's what God's Word says about laughter:

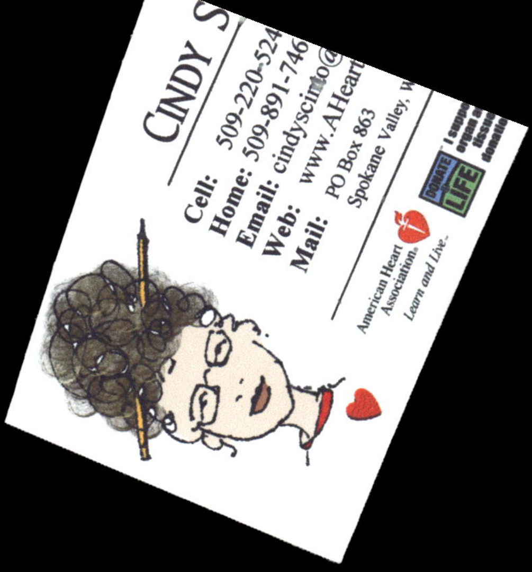

> A merry heart doeth good like a medicine (Proverbs 17:22 KJV).

> Then was our mouth filled with laughter, and our tongue with singing: then said they among the heathen, The LORD hath done great things for them" (Psalm 126: 2 KJV).

In Tim Hansel's book, *You Gotta Keep Dancin'*, laughter is hailed as paramount for making life fun. He taught a special class at Azusa Pacific University with optimum health as its focus;

> Tre was in our class. Some serious congenital problems had left her with only one leg that could do no more than hold a shoe. She had a total of six stubby fingers. But if you were to meet her, you would most likely agree with the class, [They unanimously chose Tre Bernhard as the greatest living example of wholeness that they ever knew.] because the two most predominant features about Tre are her incredible compassion and her lively sense of humor. Tre had been through hardships even worse than her physical handicaps. She had lived a life that would devastate most people, yet she chose to transcend the situation and give the world a tangible sense of love and humor that changed more than one life, including my own.
>
> Humor has the unshakable ability to break life up into little pieces and make it livable. Laughter adds richness, texture, and color to otherwise ordinary days. It is a gift, choice, a discipline, and an art.[46]

Laughter comes from a heart filled with the love of God. If you can't seem to get a good laugh going, then let me help you out. The next few stories are true—and I did not embellish them for this writing. They may not be in the order they happened, but real they are! My friends no longer say "Murphy's Law," they say it's "Cindy's Law!"

Go ahead, have a good laugh on me!

I have some one-liners most people find quite amusing. How about my reasons for still being alive? "It's too hard for them to kill me off, I'm from New York. We don't die easy!" or "I keep trying to get to heaven before everyone else, but I keep missing!"

When I finally got out of a wheelchair and onto crutches after breaking my leg, it felt good to stand—even if it was with crutches. I am only 5' 2" tall, but my remark was exasperated: "I feel so tall!"

Sometimes doctor visits can be quite amusing. One doctor in Seattle, Washington, was quite the sarcastic one. When I told him how people tell me I look great for what I have been through, his reply was, "You don't look so great to me!"

When I told him I had seen seven other cardiologists before him, he asked me, "What happened to them?"

I wanted to give him some of his own medicine back, so my reply was, "Oh, they are floating down the Spokane River by now." That stopped him from getting the last word!

Sometimes nurses at doctor's offices can be quite swirly after a long day. During one of my appointments after my heart transplant, I was belaying over my weight gain. The nurse's reply was, "At least you don't wiggle when you walk." I guess she considered me "fat but firm."

That same nurse, and I do love her, had a great idea when I broke my leg. Being on crutches made it hard to get around, and often I had to explain that I didn't break it skiing or snowboarding. I live in the snow country of Washington State, so that is a logical assumption when someone is on crutches in the winter. Her idea was almost as good as mine: "Just tell people you had a heart transplant and now you are looking for a new leg!"

Okay, I thought that was cute. Mine is a bit more of a chuckle-buster; "No, I didn't break my leg skiing. I was stealing coconuts in Florida!" (You can read about my mishap in chapter 8.)

She also referred to my unimaginable bad luck as being reminiscent to the story line in "Planes, Trains, and Automobiles" where the movie plot follows the story of character Neal Page as he tries to return to his family in Chicago for Thanksgiving after being on a business trip in New York. The journey is doomed from the outset with everything possible going wrong.

Hey, at least we can laugh!

There have also been attempts on my part to "work the system" as you might say. After being on a pacemaker for almost six months, I noticed one day that I felt more lethargic then usual. My heart rate was a steady 80 bpm. I checked it several times throughout the day and it was always 80 bpm. After a few days like this, I went in to see my cardiologist and a technician tested my pacemaker.

Everything was fine with the pacemaker, but the reason for the constant 80 bpm is that my heart was no longer beating on its own. The pacemaker had taken over entirely. I thought about that and then asked my cardiologist to make out a "death certificate." "What for?" he asked in shock.

My reply was not what he expected. "Well, if my heart is no longer beating on its own, then I am actually dead! If you make out a *death* certificate, I can send it in to my life insurance company and collect my life insurance. I could really use the money now!"

Of course, I couldn't seem to convince him!

When I had to prepare for my trip to Hershey, Pennsylvania, where I was taking part in the experimental surgery that grew new arteries around my heart, I knew my husband, son, and I were facing five weeks in a hotel.

Looking for the most economical housing, I called the Ronald McDonald House in Hershey. They told me only children and their families were able to use their facilities. My line to a newspaper reporter, which she found comical enough to use in her article about my surgery, was, "I tried to get into the Ronald McDonald House, but I was too tall!"

Speaking of accommodations, in August of 2002, when I traveled with my husband and son to New York City to have a procedure done, we had to find a hotel in Manhattan for one night. The cardiologist performing the heart catheterization did not want me to travel the very day I was discharged.

My husband tried to find a room close to the hospital, but the area of Manhattan by the hospital was very affluent and rooms were expensive. One night in a basic accommodation was no lower then $500 a night.

So he visited Hotels.com to see what he could find. He got us a room for $89 only a few blocks from the hospital.

"How did you find that deal?" I asked him as we hailed a cab.

"Oh, it was one of those specials. But at least it is close by."

We traveled the few blocks by cab so I wouldn't have to walk very far. We were dropped off in front of the hotel, its name palely displayed on an old building, "The Habitat."

"The Habitat?" I questioned. "Is that like a *hostel* for traveling students?" John was quiet as we entered the doors.

Inside we stared as employees in black clad pants and shirts waited on clients. The lobby was surreal with a mixture of modern décor and dark furnishings. To the left of the front entrance was a dance club with a disco mirror ball glaring down on dark bodies dancing to primal music.

"This is where we are staying?" I asked.

"There's nothing else around here," John replied.

We checked in and walked up a flight of stairs to an old cage-like elevator, then traveled slowly up to the sixth floor where our room was. Dingy, stained walls surrounded dark hallways as we found our room number. After opening the door and stepping in, we realized why it was so cheap.

The room was only as wide as it was deep, maybe 7 feet by 9 feet. An aged air conditioner leaned dangerously on the ledge of an old window. At least we would have cool air. Then I noticed a free-standing sink next to a small, worn-out television. "Where is the actual bathroom?" I remarked. John walked down the hall and found two bathrooms—or should I say, "toilet closets." Each was the size of an actual closet with only a toilet sitting in the middle and a light bulb in the ceiling.

"I won't use these bathrooms tonight without you guarding the door!" I nervously stated.

Now we had to find a shower—any shower. So we continued down the hallway to find a "community shower." Looking in at the tattered walls and filthy shower stalls, we decided a shower could wait until we left the next day and returned to family where we were staying.

Back to the room: I noticed there was only one twin-sized bed! John pulled it away from the wall and found that the top mattress slid out to reveal another mattress underneath. When it was fully open, it made a double bed with two mattresses. But once the bed was opened far enough for us to both sleep on it, we could no longer open the door!

"Oh, this is great," I moaned. "I can see me now having to go the bathroom tonight. I'll have to roll over you to get out of the bed, have you get up and fold up the bed, walk down the hallway hoping we don't get mugged, and then manage to use the 'toilet closet' without totally freaking out!"

We decided to make the best of it. We opened the bed, locked the door, and settled in to watch some television.

After falling asleep, like clockwork, I woke up around 2:00 a.m. to go to the bathroom. I woke up John, we rolled out of the bed, slid the top mattress back against the wall and walked down the hallway to the toilet closets. I made sure John stayed posted outside my door.

But when I was done and opened the door, he was not in the hallway. My poor heart, just being poked and prodded, started to race. "John, where are you!" I whispered as boldly as I dared.

For a scary moment, I thought he had been mugged or that I would find him down the dark hallway, murdered by an intruder.

As fast as I called out to him, he appeared, emerging from the toilet closet next to me. "What's wrong?" he chided me. "I had to use the bathroom too."

We went back to the room and the night passed with no more interruptions. I was one happy person when we checked out the next day! Don't ya love New York!

There have been other unforeseen hazards relating to my many appointments and check ups. One time, I was lying down on an exam table having a bone density test, and as it was finished, the technician tried to retract the top of it so I could sit up and get off the table. Each time she tried to retract it, it made a grinding noise and moved only an inch or so. She tried and tried, and after 10 or 15 minutes, I suggested she let me crawl out of the machine. "Oh no," she said. "That won't be okay. I don't know what is wrong. This has never happened before." She kept trying.

"Look, I am not really old with brittle bones. I can safely crawl out of this if you would let me." I definitely wanted to get out of that machine. She finally agreed and I crawled out. As I left, I could still hear the machine grinding away as she tried to unlock it.

I also have multiple visits to the lab for blood work. Sometimes I go so often I see the same lab personnel more than once in the same week. Within six months, the centrifugal machine that spins the blood sample to separate it for testing, *blew up two times* while they were spinning my blood. Blew up! Gone. The expensive machine was totally broken and had to be replaced. This can happen at times, but to happen twice within six months with *my* blood in it made the lab technicians pay attention. I wonder how they feel now when I walk in for my monthly blood work.

I've had many embarrassing moments too. I was leaving a grocery store after having a pacemaker put in to keep my heart beating properly. I had a large cart of groceries and was just going through the security screens when the alarm went off. A young store clerk came over to check my cart. He looked and looked, but couldn't find anything with a security tag on it. Finally I told him I had a pacemaker. He felt silly and walked away quietly. I, of course, felt just as silly that I was so young looking, he never thought of me having a pacemaker!

I've met some pretty special people since getting sick. One such person, Michelle, has gone through much—if not more—than I have. We used to get together and whine about our situations, but sometimes the whining gave way to creative laughter.

Before my transplant, while I was still able to drive, Michelle called asked me if I could take her to her heart catheterization—part of the yearly checkup a transplant patient must go through to keep tabs on their new heart. She was scheduled for early in the morning—very early, but I knew she needed someone not only to drive her, but also to be with her.

The day before, I had my pacemaker adjusted. My "sleeping" heart was totally dependent on the device for the electrical impulses it needed to keep beating. Most of the time, I was very tired from all the medications, machines, and appointments I faced. Four a.m. would be early! But she needed to be at the hospital by 5:00 a.m..

I woke up to my alarm that Thursday with a groggy murmur. When I got to Michelle's, she was waiting at the door. We got in my van and headed out. While driving on the highway, to the hospital, I had a disconcerting idea.

"You know, if one of us has a heart attack, the other will have a heart attack from the emotional stress. So who will call 911? Look at us; it's the blind leading the blind!"

We laughed all the rest of the way to the hospital!

¤ ¤ ¤

I know I have told you about having been an inpatient at my local hospital more then 55 times. So if you really fathom that, I had many opportunities to experience everyday hospital mishaps. Of course, someone visiting a few times over many years may never fall into some of the *silly* things that happen, but with my frequent visits, you know things are going to go awry.

Early on in my *heart catheterization career*, I learned about the aftermath of such a procedure. A heart cath, or angioplasty, is an exploratory and/or intervention procedure performed by a cardiologist to diagnose and repair heart blockages or other abnormalities. Because the procedure involves sending a wire up through the femoral artery in your groin area, you must lie flat for a period of time after the procedure so that the artery can heal without bleeding. A femoral artery bleed can be fatal.

The amount of time you lie flat can vary from one hour for just a diagnostic procedure up to 18 hours for an interventional procedure. At one time, after one heart cath led to another one the same afternoon, I maxed out at 36 hours lying flat! When I was granted privileges to vacate my hospital bed, I ran for the bathroom, locked myself in, and wouldn't come out for an hour. I did not want to see another bedpan and I just wanted the freedom to say, "Stay away from me!"

Okay, my first heart cath was traumatic with the doctors trying to avoid open-heart surgery or death. I don't even remember how long I had to lie flat then. But consider this: lying flat after this procedure means (and some of you may have been here already) FLAT. No moving any body part except for your arms. No moving your legs, unless you have permission to wiggle the opposite leg a bit, no moving your torso, and absolutely *no* picking up your head to see beyond your nose!

After you are given these instructions and told to ring the call light if you have to use the bedpan (and you will have to use it frequently due to the fluids they push through your veins to help your kidneys), you are then granted a food tray. Having been NPO (nothing per mouth) for hours, you find yourself very hungry. If the kitchen gets it right, the food tray sent up should consist of finger-friendly foods—food that can be eaten from a prone position *easily* with your fingers.

The second heart cath to repair a blockage opened up a new world for me. I never thought I would become an expert at handling the aftermath. I was brought back to my room and "slid" back onto my bed. Given the instructions once more, I buckled down for an eight-hour session of flatness. The nurse handed me my call button and told me the kitchen was sending up a tray of food. I was relieved the worse was over and looking forward to some substance for my grumbling stomach.

The food tray arrived pretty fast and the food service worker set it on my bed table, aligning it so I could reach the contents. She left and I uncovered the plate. Under that brown, airtight, insulated top was a bowl—a bowl of steaming hot soup! How did they expect me to eat soup? There was a spoon on the tray, the nurses were in the middle of shift change, and I was hungry. So spoon in hand I dipped into the soup and guided it to my mouth, trying to keep a flat angle. I carefully lowered the spoon over my mouth, but the soup dribbled down my neck leaving behind bits of carrots and celery, not to mention the uncomfortable sensation of a wet hospital gown and pillowcase. After a few attempts, a nurse came in and was surprised at my dilemma.

"Why did they give you soup?" she exclaimed. "I'll call down to get you another tray with finger food."

"Thank you," was my reply. I hoped it wouldn't take too long.

Another tray of food was delivered. By now my doctor had come in to check on me. She was my endocrinologist and was concerned about my blood sugar levels and hospital diet. Now remember, I was in a room on the Advanced Cardiac Unit.

After chatting a bit, she said, "Here, why don't I help you with your food? Hopefully this time it won't be soup!" She uncovered the plate of food and we both stared in shock. Under that insulated, plastic, brown, cover was a gigantic mound of FRENCH FRIES! Soggy, greasy, French fries! We both stared in shock. How could they serve French fries on a cardiac unit to a diabetic and in such a large quantity?

Of course she had the nurse come in and retrieve the tray. "When we order finger food for a heart patient, we don't mean French fries," was her response. "Please order another tray with appropriate food."

Once again the kitchen was contacted to send up the right food. One other thing I always do in the hospital is order a vegetarian diet. Not because I am a full-time vegetarian, but have you noticed what kind of "meat" they serve in a hospital? Known as mystery meat, I prefer not to even have to smell it arriving in my room.

So, another tray comes up, and they tried to accommodate me being vegetarian. But the only thing on the tray was a bunch of cut up carrots and celery—and nothing else. I was hoping for maybe some cheese or, hey, a sandwich be a novel idea. When the nurse saw the meager vegetables, she asked me what I wanted to do. "Tell them I am a vegetarian but I don't want just vegetables. Ask them to send me a vegetarian tray with more than just vegetables."

Up comes the last tray. The nurse brings it in with four of her colleagues following her in a procession. Everyone wanted to see what was going to be under the cover this time. Someone hummed a drum roll. The food was placed on my bed table. I stared intensely at the tray. My right arm reached over to grab the cover. All eyes were on the plate and, in one swoop, I lifted the cover and there was, to everyone's shock, a large, heaping plate of MIXED vegetables, cooked and piled high. I was so done. I wanted no more attempts from the kitchen! I called my dear friend Terry and begged her to bring me some real food. She arrived 30 minutes later with tacos. I ate it without guilt. After all, the hospital food was going to either kill me or starve me!

Lesson learned—bring your own food if you are admitted to a hospital! But . . . be very careful about how you sneak forbidden food in!

Terry, being one of my faithful friends who has gone beyond comprehensible limits to help me in any way, was famous for bringing items like Dairy Queen's peanut buster parfait or once in a while a good, old-fashioned cheeseburger and French fries. I had my share of healthy food—so occasionally a little junk food was good for my morale! Normally, if she brought me a peanut buster parfait, she could sneak it in pretty easily. All I had to do was bury the empty container deep enough in the garbage pail and brush my teeth to get rid of the smell of ice cream on my breath.

On one occasion, however, as I craved some cholesterol, Terry brought me a cheeseburger and fries. As careful as she tried to be, the hospital chaplain for the cardiac floor saw her deliver the goods to my room. Immediately, he ran to my dietician to blab about my altercation. From then on, Terry would disguise my booty in a gift bag sealed in a plastic Ziploc!

What about embarrassing moments throughout the many inpatient visits? You will laugh—or maybe cry. Like the flying bedpan story. (Those of you who are squeamish should skip the next paragraph.)

I am lying flat after one of my many heart caths and it came time to use the bedpan. Hospitals have some odd idea that their "new" bedpans are more efficient. Maybe for storage, but the new, plastic ones are way too small. So I always ask for the old fashioned metal bedpan. This one time, I had a nurse's aide who wasn't familiar with my routine. The other aide would sprinkle some powder on the metal bedpan to avoid it sticking to me. This aide could not find any powder and offered some hand cream.

"I'm not sure that is a good idea," I cautioned.

"Oh, it will work fine," she replied confidently. I wasn't worried about it *not* working, but actually working *too* well. So she placed the bedpan, coated with hand cream, under my body. Within a second of me lying back on it, the metal pan slid out from under me and went *flying* through the air, past her and my husband, and hit the wall. After it crashed to the floor, we all looked for a moment and then burst out laughing. A bit of advice—no hand cream on a bedpan!

Then there are roommates and occupants adjacent to the hospital rooms I occupied. Since my heart transplant, I am confined to a private, germ-free, isolation room. But before that I had some roommates I played antics with. After a while, that earned me a private room and usually the one right across from the nurse's station where they could keep an eye on me.

During one of my earlier visits, I had a roommate, close to my age, who wasn't morbidly ill, but was recovering from a heart procedure. Hating the humiliating hospital gowns they give you to wear, she wanted to get a set of "scrubs" to wear instead. (Scrubs consist of a top and pants and are not issued to the patients. They are highly sought after when you are stuck in a hospital for a while.)

"Don't worry, Theresa, I will get you some scrubs."

"How?" she asked me.

"Just watch." I pressed the call button and my nurse came by to see what I needed.

"Can I help you, Cindy?" he asked? "He" was Mark, a tall, good-looking RN with a great personality.

"Yeah, can you send in Laura?" Laura was another nurse who had worked with me on a previous visit. Mark looked puzzled but sent her in. I whispered something in her ear and she looked at me like I was crazy.

"Do you know how hard it is to get those? I can't even get a set if I wanted them for myself, let alone a patient!" She turned around and stormed out, yelling back that she would see what she could do.

Theresa asked me how I got to her to try. "Oh, I have some dirt on her that wouldn't sit well with the head nurse," I told her. "She will get us the scrubs or I will have to turn her in." Theresa looked bewildered. I smirked at the joy of such mischief.

Not an hour later, Laura was back with two, neatly wrapped, freshly cleaned sets of scrubs. She threw them down on my bed. "Here, am I free now?" she snapped at me with a hint of a smile on her lips.

"Okay, you're off the hook. Just don't let anyone in here while we change!"

I went over to Theresa's bed and started to help her change into her scrubs. It was crazy to get the top and pants on with all the tubing and IVs she was hooked up to. She was getting out of breath and I was worried she might have another heart attack! "Maybe I should give this up," I said. "You're having a hard time breathing!"

"Oh no," she replied, "I am so excited to have these instead of that terrible gown. I am not giving them up now!"

I got her all dressed and back in her bed. Just as I started getting out of my gown and into my set of scrubs, Mark walked back in. There I was with the pants halfway up and the shirt entangled in my IV tubing.

"What in the world are you doing? And where did you get those scrubs? And why is your roommate's heart rate so fast?" Trying to answer without laughing so hard, I told him I made a deal with someone to get us scrubs. Of course I wouldn't tell him who. Nor would Theresa or I give up our scrubs. He was so mad!

We both stayed in those scrubs for three days. We finally stank so bad we had to give them up. But for a time, we had a small piece of victory and independence! Tip: You may have to wear a hospital gown because of all the tubing they poke into you, but at least bring your own underwear and pajama pants!

So many long hours were spent in my hospital room that I became very creative with projects to keep myself busy. At one point, I satisfied the urge to better the stay for other patients by creating a David Letterman-type list to distribute to those whose hospital stay extended out beyond a tolerant limit:

The Top Ten Reasons You Know You've Been in the Hospital Too Long

10

You press the call button and instead of "Can I help you?" the nurse asks on a first name basis, "Can I help you, Judy . . .?"

9

You hope to graduate from a bed-pan to a bedside commode so you can have your very own personal roll of toilet paper.

8

The lab technician flicks on the lights at 4:00 a.m. and you're sitting up in bed with your arm outstretched and fist clenched tightly.

7

The bell signaling food service is on the floor, causing a mad rush to clear your bedside tray and return your pillows to an upright position.

6

The sound of the shower running in the room next to you triggers severe jealousy as you sponge bath yourself in hopes of one day gaining the privilege of a real shower.

5

When the volunteer comes around with a cart full of activities and reading materials, you choose a "bored" game to play with your invisible friend.

4

During the half hour of Bingo on the hospital's TV channel, you refuse all treatments or nursing requests as you frantically search for G57.

3

You keep a chart to calculate how many turkey sandwiches the hospital serves per day.

2

You recognize the nurse's footsteps—and time it just right so that you can salt your mashed potatoes and hide the saltshaker before she comes back.

1

And—The Number 1 Reason You Know You've Been in the Hospital Too Long:

You open the small closet in your room and an
avalanche of packaged saltine crackers, graham
crackers, and packets of salt and sugar you collected
come tumbling down on your head!

So there have actually been funny sides to all the painful times. And my lasting legacy is a befitting title assigned to me by one of the transport personnel at the hospital. I had an alternate ego that I appropriately displayed with a gold tiara, red cloak, and jeweled sceptre. Whenever I was allowed to walk the hallways on the cardiac unit, I placed my tiara on my head, draped my red, silk cape over my drab hospital gown, and toted my sceptre, being sure to knight whomever I saw in the hallways. It worked great when I was in the hospital for Halloween on several occasions.

One time when I was walking about, I spotted an unknown doctor at the nurse's station. Walking up to him with royal flare, I used my sceptre to knight him and declared him "Sir Doctor." He turned pale, slowly backed up, and made his way to the elevators. I guess he didn't have a sense of humor. Well, you gotta' laugh!

Chapter 7
I Am Who I Am

"You will be trading one set of problems for another, but you will be alive." That is the proclamation I received from my heart transplant coordinator and my surgeon. Somehow I felt like they rehearsed the same line so they could deliver it to each person who was lucky enough to receive a life-saving heart transplant.

When I first heard these words, I was so desperately fighting for my life, I didn't care what trade-off I had to make. I just wanted to live. But one day, while on line at the airport to board a plane, a young girl asked me a poignant question. She noticed I was wearing a face mask, something I must wear when I travel by plane. She also noticed a sign I was wearing around my neck. I made it in defiance of the stares and comments I receive anytime I travel. It had a heart and a stethoscope with the words, "Heart Transplant—Germs make me sick" printed out in big red letters. (I am finally over the phobia and now travel without a "label.")

"Did you ever feel like you would have rather died?" she asked. "I mean, if I was in your situation, I think I would rather have died than to live with all the hassles you endure. I am not married and don't have any children, so I guess it makes a difference."

She showed a genuine interest and her question was honest and viable. But it dumbfounded me. I didn't know what to say. Her question made me consider what I go through every day and how my life and who I am has changed so much. Here I was traveling with the rest of the world and still I have to wear a mask marking me as different and, to some people, marking me as a possible threat. In fact, quite often, someone will inevitably decide I am some contagious creature and change their seat, avoid me, cover their own face, or ask something insulting.

When you first receive an organ transplant, you are more susceptible to germs, and the rest of your life you will be "immune suppressed," or living with an immune system that is almost completely turned off. For the first three to six months, anywhere you go outside of your own home is dangerous so you must wear a face mask. I received some of the harshest reactions from people in grocery stores, department stores, restaurants, and anywhere I went in public. I must say though, sometimes it got me a better seat as no one would sit next to me. Or, I would go to the front of the line when checking out in a store.

One time, when I was in line in a grocery store at the deli counter, a woman asked me if I had anything that was contagious. I told her I had had a heart transplant and was not supposed to be exposed to germs so I had to wear the mask for protection. She never heard what I said; she just stayed focused on the mask. "But I don't want to get sick," she clamored. "I just can't get sick." She was frantic about getting sick.

"I am not sick," I reassured her. Still she left the line with her hand over her mouth and even left the store. I went up to the counter to place my order and the deli clerk smiled.

"I guess it can come in handy—having a heart transplant." I smirked at the absurdity of it.

Would I have rather died than go through a heart transplant? I answered the question coming from the girl in the airport after a minute or so, but wasn't sure I was even convinced. "Well, I have a husband and a teenage son who need me. I wanted to be here for them." She looked at me quizzically and pondered my answer.

"I guess that makes sense," she replied. We boarded the plane and I still consider her question. Sometimes I am so worn-out from all the health problems, appointments, insurance claims and hassles, medications and their side effects, not being able to physically do things I like, daily struggles, and the ominous shadow of my shortened lifespan, that I waver a bit on my decision to choose to live. But the thought is immediately snuffed out when I think of how selfish that would be to want to avoid all the struggles and leave behind no good testimony of what God can do when we trust Him for each day's battle. Although I am different physically, I am still who I am.

Becoming a Christian sometimes terrified me. I often worried about how to change who I was and what I was. I internalized much about myself and scurried around utilizing way too many "sharp edges" to do my own pruning in hope of being the *best* Christian I could be.

God got a hold of me on certain occasions and He has a way of taking sometimes the quietest moment, the simplest environment, and using the time to make a tremendous statement. One warm, summer night on Lake Coeur d'Alene in Idaho, He did just that.

The crescent moon hung low in the dark evening sky amid stars positioned in their appointed places. A caressing breeze rippled over the deck as our cruise ship meandered along the velvet, peaceful lake. I looked around through dimly lit groups of people—some were sitting and singing as praise and worship choruses undulated from the musicians at the bow of the ship. Others stood, faces towards the horizon and hands raised in peaceful worship. The evening was surreal.

The melodic phrases of Amazing Grace were being sung when suddenly, lights appeared in the sky—the Northern Lights. Colors danced and shifted against the black sky as nature's light show hung down like majestic draperies. The Northern Lights can only be seen at certain times of the year and conditions must be just right for them to appear. I had always wanted to witness their unearthly phenomenon, and for most, the appearance of such a natural wonder was the perfect ending to a perfect evening.

But as I stood in the midst of all this splendor, tears streamed down my cheeks. I was struggling to hold back a torrent of weeping emotions. The ship, a dinner cruise reserved for our church group, held four hundred people and both top and bottom decks were filled. With people all around me, there was nowhere to escape. I tried my hardest to hide the pain that was trying to gush forth from inside my tormented soul. What was a beautiful evening for most became the finalization of a work the Lord started in me years before. I arrived, that night, at the furthest point of control—the emptiest part of my own self-realization.

Leaving the ship, I made it to our car without anyone noticing how much I had cried. I looked over at my husband and asked, "How do you know when you've had an emotional breakdown?" He looked at me, puzzled by the abrupt question.

"Why do you ask?"

"I think I had one tonight." My reply was straight-out. The rest of the drive home was in silence. But once we got our son to bed and sat down with a cup of tea, the tears began and I sobbed the innermost nuggets of pain from my broken heart. All the issues from my past—that is, my past as a Christian, which I believed I took control of and rid myself of—were being paraded in front of me one by one. The Lord seemed to grab each circumstance and hold it up to my face, letting me know there was trash I was holding on to tightly. For the first time, I could clearly see my problem with control. I sought to control my life, my spiritual state, my circumstances, my purpose, and even my destiny. For someone who thought they had let go of all control, I now realized I was safely hiding the last fragments of my own domination.

What I did with many issues throughout the years was to conquer them on my own and neatly tuck them away. The problem with such annihilation is that a complete ridding of bitterness, scars, anger, sin, unforgiveness, and other roots of hurt cannot happen unless the Lord gets complete control. I read all the scriptures about forgiveness. I paid attention to the many deep sermons on "letting go" and profusely studied how to grow close enough to the Lord to let Him control my life. When I confidently awarded myself with an A+ for passing the school of letting go, He stripped me down to bare my soul and expose my folly.

Where did the intense desire to control my life come from? I can see the dynamite in memories as far back as my childhood.

¤ ¤ ¤

"Let go of her, Laura, or I'll deck you one." My voice was strengthened with anger and vengeance as I lunged toward the assailant. Laura's fists were swinging as she aimed at Sara, a much smaller and younger girl. Being a tomboy and bully, Laura could easily inflict the harm she intended on her victim. "Oh no, you don't," I asserted as I grabbed Laura's neck and yanked her off Sara.

Turning Laura around, I pinned her against the wall of our cabin and began to hurl punches at her—hitting and missing in my moment of fury. Her feet dangled off the wooden floor as she struggled to get free of my grip. Considering I was much smaller than her, it was amazing that I could keep her prisoner to my attack.

"Cynthia! What on earth are you doing to that poor girl?" I can still hear the exasperated yell of the camp counselor. She pulled me away as Laura's body sunk to the floor. Huddled in a bundle of tears, Laura pointed at me, yelling out in anger that I had started the whole fight.

We were both marched to the main office where a senior counselor ironed out the truth and instructed us to hug and make up. Hours later, Laura was planning another assault while the rest of us sang around a roasting campfire. I watched my back in anticipation of a secret attack.

I was only ten years old when I first realized the power of my anger and wrath and the unending desire to control what surrounded me. Being raised with 12 siblings in New York, combined with the velocity of an Italian heritage, destined me to be a neatly packaged stick of dynamite. Wholehearted causes, arguments, the need for survival and everyday struggles of life in a large family bred the instinct to control and shape my surroundings.

My husband, barely 17 when I latched onto him, became the object of my desire to gain control and comfort. I looked to him to fulfill my shortcomings—the areas where I had no reins to steer and direct.

We married six years after John first asked me to go steady. Our relationship appeared to be the perfect courtship. Even the circumstances for his proposal were cleverly manipulated by my need to move out from the clutches of my home life. I became the decision maker and controller. I did not allow my husband to take his place as spiritual leader and head of my household. Overwhelmed by my dominating design, he became reclusive, leaving me to deal with all matters of our marriage. It made for an unbalanced and insecure relationship.

When our son came along and financial and medical problems mounted, I demanded that John step in and fix everything. But I had created a lopsided relationship that needed drastic measures to be righted. With much heartbreak, we sought the help of a Christian counselor. After several sessions, this gentle, gracious counselor looked at me with intent and said, "You have to let go of your desire to control everything. Let your husband be who he needs to be in this marriage." I was instantly deflated. Had I really taken control? Hadn't I given up the old me a long time ago when I asked Jesus to be my Lord? No, there was much more to the cleansing than I could ever foresee. This was merely a small advance to be rid of a deep-rooted cause.

I have learned that many times when we struggle with an area of our lives that we cannot overcome, giving it to the Lord may entail a multifaceted process. Our Lord is a creative God who knows each of us intimately. If we allow Him to be the One who conquers our hurdle, it will be complete—He will not leave a trace to take root and become an issue for us again. God's cleansing is complete and perfect.

In my mind, I can still see the Northern Lights from that evening. They spread their color and radiated through the black sky dotted with stars. After twenty minutes or so, they blended softly into the dark horizon.

I can be who I am. My identity is not lost in Christ but celebrated through Him. There is much power in a person who is not in control. Opposite as it may be to the world's thinking, there is One who can do a much better job at leading our lives through the foreign world we live in. When I was a young girl, I dreamed of becoming the first woman president. And I am—president of my place in God's perfect plan for my life. I sit at the top with His arm over my shoulder, pointing out the glorious way He has put together my days.

I often think of how many times I avoided meeting new people after I got sick. I didn't want anyone to know the "new" me. I wanted them to know who I was and what I could do before heart disease crippled me. I was afraid I had lost the person I was to someone who was disabled and trodden down. I no longer had the qualities I once possessed. It took me a long time to emerge from my own ashes and peek out at a different life ahead of me. I am still struggling to resist the desire to hide from the world.

In the February 2008 edition of the AHA's *Heart Insight Magazine*, Kathleen Prentice writes about how her life changed after surviving an unexpected heart attack while caring for her children and aging parents. She titles one section in her article "When a Caregiver Needs Care" as *The New Normal* and writes:

> My life had changed from being a biker and swimmer to feeling grateful to be able to walk from the sofa to the shower by myself, grateful to be home, grateful to be alive, grateful to share a laugh with my daughter.... I felt like I had relinquished control over my job description, my identity.... I had to accept letting Bob, Caitlin and younger daughter, Lily, take over the household and my care—and to accept how they did it.... What I wanted most of all, was to return to normal. What we've ended up with is a blend of pre-and-post heart attack routines. A new normal.[47]

A *new normal* is not always what we want normal to be. So many things can change and our lives can become a state of bedlam. After one of my many ER visits, my son, then 13 years old and in the middle of his teen years, stated "This is never going to end, is it?" His normal was long gone. I picked him up from school one day and after seeing a failing test grade, I asked him "What do you think about all day, Jonathan?"

His answer broke my already frail heart, "Mom, I never know if you are going to be dead or alive when I get home from school." His view of me took on a very different form.

Look at how normal was forever changed for Joni Eareckson-Tada in her book, *Joni*. Many of you may remember her story. In 1967, Joni, a teenager enjoying summer break, suffered a diving accident that left her paralyzed from the neck down. Her ministry,

Joni and Friends, has since touched people with or without disabilities all over the world.

I remember one section of her book where she came to terms with struggling with her self-image.

> I'd still look at healthy, active people—attractive people—enjoying themselves around me. Everyone I compared myself to came out best. I'd even lose out when I compared myself to a mannequin!
>
> Her friend Steve answered her quandary, "But that's the same for everyone if we let society determine our value. We always lose if we evaluate ourselves according to someone else's ideas or standards. And there are as many standards as there are people. We have to forget about what people say or think and recognize that God's values are the only important ones."
>
> It was true. God knew that I had hands and feet and arms and legs that did not work. He knew what I looked like. And none of these things really mattered. What counted was that I was His workmanship created in His image. And He wasn't finished with me. (Eph. 2:10)[48]

"He wasn't finished with me." Joni's words make me think of how often I wanted to go back to being the "old" me. But that is just what the past is—old, and I needed, and still need, to realize I am "new." I am a new person with new direction.

One day I met someone who has forever changed my life and caused me to keep my eyes off the past.

I was at the hospital, having yet another heart catheterization. John was there along with a few other people who were visiting and offering encouragement. One of the pastors from our church showed up and said he wanted us to meet someone. I looked out in the hallway, and there was Jeff. He wheeled in with his motorized wheelchair and a big, sunny smile on his face. The drab room lit up with his joyful presence.

Jeff was there to pray for me and to offer his support in any way he could. The last thing I remember before I was wheeled to the operating room was Jeff talking with John. His face watched and pondered as John spoke to him and it was clear he was interested in John—interested in how he was doing. I was content to see someone there for John, not just me.

Soon after that first meeting, Jeff "typed" me an email. I emphasize "typed" as Jeff's wheelchair confinement is due to the loss of both his arms and the use of his legs in an electrocution accident several years prior when he was just 30 years old. He types with the ends of each "claw" attached where his hands should be. It's a long process for him to get through typing even one page.

Jeff was a successful business owner, maintaining billboards, and had a family of five children, the youngest being only 13 days old. It was a week before Christmas and Jeff was singing Christmas carols, thinking of bringing his children to visit Santa. He was up on a billboard, 40 feet high, when his equipment came into contact with an electrical line that was out of place. Over 14,400 bolts of electricity burned through his body, and he was killed instantly.

But as he fell to the ground, the jolt started his heart back up. He died again several times but, by a miracle, lived through the first few days when he was not expected to make it. The ensuing year was spent in painful rehabilitation. As it now stands, he has limited use of his battered legs, he wears two prosthetic arms with claws, controlled by straps attached to his back, and he endures severe pain every moment of each day and long night. Below is his letter to me, typed in his own words back in November of 2003.

Dear Cindy,

Don't you just hate being a human...I know that I do sometimes! I went through that a little bit...with we're going to cut this off....No, we're going to try and save it...many times over. Like you, I'm a pretty positive person...and ultimately trust God and His will....Unfortunately I had my down times, troubled times, and angry times...And that hellish roller coaster ride just consumed me, and prolonged the bad times, so that they were outnumbering and outlasting the positive times. This is what I ultimately decided...and it may not be for you...it just worked for me. I took all of the trust and hope that I had placed in docs, circumstances, luck, and my own strength...and cleared it out.

I also had several weeks with a life-threatening infection near my spine...They tried everything, they were opening me up at least once a week and cutting away the infected tissue...I was on the most powerful antibiotic known to man...nothing was working...it looked like the infection was going to be fatal. I know that it probably sounds morbid...it does to me...as I type...but I went ahead and said Lord, it doesn't look like I'll make it...please give me peace about dying...I would just ask that you use me until then. It worked!

I read a lot of Paul's writings...We can both relate to him...I played a couple of songs frequently...my favorite was "My Hope Is In You" ...by 3rd day...Eventually they put antibiotic beads near my spine, and I got through it. I made my peace with losing ALL of my limbs, at the torso...When they stopped at an elbow, and just below my shoulder...I was thrilled! Even though they had hopes (which were contagious) of preserving more. At least for me...I was still able to be positive...because I was vigilantly watching for that one opportunity where God could use me...

I didn't get pre-occupied with death, or dwell on it...I just made the most of the time I had with my family...I didn't tell them about my mind-set...they wouldn't have understood...and would have thought that I was throwing in the towel, and been hurt and upset. They would have spent all of our time together trying to talk me out of my new perspective.

The bottom line is that God honored it...He did use me, and He was glorified. So now...any development short of death...doesn't surprise me...No, I'm not the picture of joy that I think Paul was...but it enables me to deal with it nonetheless....

After my accident, when I woke up after eight days...I realized that I had a big house payment, a mini-van payment, and two truck payments from my business...no savings, no disability, and putrid medical insurance...five young kids to feed...It was way beyond me...it was totally hopeless for me...so I had no option other than giving it ALL completely over to God...He handled everything in His timing...paid off the vehicles, and then the house...with less than $500 left over...it was beautiful.

I really was fortunate...because I could've/would've worked out a plan if it was humanly possible...after all, I worked harder than anyone I knew. I was a successful businessman, I even built my own home...If anyone could do it...I could. My situation was so ridiculously impossible...I didn't have a choice...but I did have a prayer...a prayer of desperation and faith...God rose to the challenge, and met our needs in such a miraculous way...that it affected hundreds of people...and still does when I tell my story to a group...it literally changed people's lives.

I can honestly say, Cindy...that if I was in a similar situation as you guys (I don't know everything) but a scenario in which there was a glimmer of hope...I wouldn't have been able to give it to God 100%...I would have missed the miracle and blessing...and so would have hundreds...maybe thousands of others. So I just want to encourage you to relax...spend some time reminding yourself of God's promises...I'm in this with you guys for the looong haul...eternity. I am blessed and encouraged immeasurably by spending time with you.

I pray for you guys every time God puts you on my heart...I imagine that those are the down times for you...anyway...I'm wearing out the sharp end of my hook with all of this typing....

Love you guys,
Jeff [49]

Here is Jeff, a young man with so much life to live and so much to look forward to and now he can only look forward to getting through each day. His youthful body, now prisoner to the physical trauma, drains his days with pain and helplessness. People stare at the plastic replacements for his hard-working, muscular arms and the claws that act as hands. But Jeff keeps his sense of humor, offering opening lines like, “Hi, I’m Jeff. Shake my claw!”

Does the appearance of Jeff change who he is? People will look at him with pre-existing ideas of his worth. But Jeff is stronger and better then he ever was. His worth to God is more valuable with a broken body as long as his heart is sustained only by God’s power.

A similar story of visible transformation occurred for Greg Gadson. Gadson, a brawny, determined athlete for the Army football team, was returning from memorial services for two soldiers from his battalion when a roadside bomb hit the truck he was traveling in. A lieutenant colonial in the Army's Warrior Transition Brigade, Gadson lost both his legs in the accident, and would never play football again. Though he faced life from the sidelines, physically, it did not stop him from being a team player and being given credit for leading the New York Giants to a Super Bowl victory in 2007.

A former school mate at West Point, now a coach for the New York Giants, went to see Gadson in the hospital:

> The coach watched as Gadson interacted with the other patients and the doctors and nurses, encouraging them all. "To see the impact he had on these people—the look in his eyes and how they responded—was overwhelming and inspirational."
>
> When the Giants were scheduled to play the Redskins in Washington three months later, Sullivan [the coach] sent his friend tickets—along with a request: Would Gadson speak to the team before they took the field? Having lost the first two games of the season, the Giants had already given up 80 points and, worse, seemed to be playing with no heart. The coach felt that Gadson was the perfect person to tell the players something they needed to hear about commitment, about perseverance, about teamwork.
>
> The Giants were a losing team until Gadson gave them the heart to win.[50]

It is people like Gadson who can tell their story of tragedy and instill the desire in others to grow into who God made them to be.

In the fall of 1974, Tim Hansel, went from a healthy, strong, vibrant lifestyle to one of constant pain after his climbing accident. Tim relates to the tragedy of losing who he was and living with pain and constraints on a daily basis. He took sage advice from his doctor and found himself finally free to be who he was made to be by God;

> "Son, listen to me carefully. The damage has been done. My recommendation is that you live your life as fully and richly as possible. Bite the bullet and live to be a hundred. As far as I can tell, you can do whatever the pain will allow you to do." I left with a new lease on life, a resurgent hope for the future, and a new commitment to live life again with a sense of abandonment.
>
> As strange as it may seem, up to that point I hadn't known I had a choice. I had allowed myself to step into the victim mentality without wanting it or knowing it. But through a gentle doctor, our Lord again "turned my mourning into dancing, and my sackcloth into joy" (Psalm 30:11).[51]

A friend once asked me how I was able to stay as upbeat as I was and keep my personality intact after all that I suffered and continued to suffer. My reply was a simple numerical value: -0-. I had to get myself out of the way and make myself a -0- and let God be 100 percent of my strength. No, I did not lose who I was or become incapable of fighting for myself. But the only fighting I had to do was to "fight" off "self."

"God is in the midst of her, she will not be moved" (Psalm 46:5 NASB). As long as God makes up 100% of me, I shall not be moved by whatever comes at me. There's a pain scale used in all hospitals and clinics called the "Faces of Pain." The numbers to rate your pain go from zero to ten with ten being the worst. I like to think of the scale as my *self meter*. When my *self* is at a zero, I am joyful and happy because God is in complete control. When my *self* is at ten, the joy is gone as I have taken the control away from God and tried to get through the pain without Him.

I now have a new physical heart, but its life expectancy is more unsure than most people's hearts. This new heart beats with distrustful promise of supporting my body's demand for blood and oxygen—the life flow it needs to survive. Yet I must solely lean on God to provide my every breath. I constantly evaluate each moment and regard my life as one that belongs to God. Surrendered to His will for my life, I give God all that He wants—the "I am" of my soul, the all of my spiritual heart. I am still who I am even though people may judge me physically or by my abilities. God molded me into who I am meant to be. He must be at the top of my scale.

As I waited for a donor heart to become available, I often wondered about who might end up being the donor. Knowing someone had to die in order for me to live placed an awkward stigma on desiring a life-saving transplant. And part of the strangeness was the feeling of having someone else's heart beating inside of me. It comes to me as a much venerated occurrence.

Charles Siebert, a medical writer who frequently contributes to the *New York Times Magazine,* writes the following after attending a party held for more than one hundred heart transplant recipients:

> All the people I met at the party spoke in the same reverent tones about the angel in their chests, about this gift, this responsibility they now bear, and the little prayer they say to the other person inside of them.[52]

My heart donor was known to me only as a 28-year-old girl. Because of privacy and respect, the donor and recipient families are protected from being contacted by each other's families and friends. But as the recipient, I was allowed to write a letter signed with my first name only and not to include any other details of my identity. An office representing the organ donation foundation where the donor lived would deliver the letter to the appropriate donor family member.

I wrote a letter three months after my transplant. It was very difficult to know what to say. I kept it short, mailed it, and prayed and hoped for a chance to get to know more about my donor. As Siebert states in his article, there is a reverence for the person whose heart now beats in your chest. I felt a connection to whoever this girl was and had a strong yearning to meet her family—whoever they were.

Time went by, then one Friday I was led to call the organ donor organization and see if they thought it would be imposing to write another letter. The coordinator was shocked to hear from me that particular day. "Your donor's mom just called a couple of days ago to see if she could find out how the person was who had gotten her daughter's heart," she told me.

"Do you think she may want to be in touch?" I asked with hesitation.

"It's a good sign," she reassured me. "I will call her and let you know."

I hung up the phone and cried. "She has a mom," I kept walking around saying. "My donor has a mom." Just knowing someone was out there and connected to the heart beating in my chest gave me a whole new feeling of urgency to know who they were. I knew I had an extended family somewhere.

That next Monday, the coordinator called me. "Charlotte," my donor's mom, wanted to get in touch! And her daughter's name whose heart was beating in my chest was "Danielle." She told me she would be sending the permission papers to both of us to fill out and sign, and then we were free to contact each other. I was thrilled and excited about the chance to know more about Danielle's family.

In time, I began to talk with Charlotte on the phone. We cried mostly, laughed at similarities between her daughter and me, and finally planned to meet on Easter weekend. I learned that Danielle had three brothers and a stepdad. I also got to know Danielle and what led up to the tragic accident that took her life away but gave me mine back.

When Danielle was five years old, her dad was killed in a motorcycle accident leaving Charlotte to raise three children on her own. They often had to visit the local food bank to get help with the growing family's needs. Danielle was so touched by the act of kindness, she insisted to her mom that when she grew up she would "help others like they were helping them." And as she grew, she did just that—gave whatever she had if someone she saw needed it. She gave her coat away to a friend and came home in the cold rain without it; her shoes were donated to a friend in need as she walked home barefoot; her lunch was often offered to another classmate who had nothing; and she always asked for extra snacks to hand out to those less fortunate.

As she got older, Danielle explained to her mom that she felt like she was put on the earth to give to those who were in need of help. When she got her drivers license, she decided to become an organ donor. "Mom, if something were to happen to me, why would I want my organs to be buried when someone's life could be saved or helped by me being a donor?"

No one likes to talk about a subject as sensitive as dying, but it was important to Danielle that her family knew her wishes. Still, the tragic day came when as Charlotte put it, "I lost something very dear to me—my little princess."

Danielle was an epileptic and had a seizure one day that caused her to slip and fall in the shower. She suffered a concussion and also hit her nec, cutting off blood flow to her brain from her carotid arteries in her neck. After three days in the hospital, all hope was lost that she would ever come back. When Charlotte was notified that the hospital called a code blue on Danielle, the acronym for eminent death, she was distraught. "Why God, why are you doing this? Take me instead of her."

Danielle's brothers and the rest of her family all struggled with their loss. But Charlotte knew that God had a purpose on earth for her daughter—her "princess." She also knew that if Danielle's organs had not been donated, there would have been no purpose to her death.

The holidays were always difficult for Charlotte, but after talking for a few months, she agreed to meet my family and I on Easter weekend, almost three years after losing Danielle. It was an emotional and powerful meeting for both of us—Charlotte finding closure and me getting to know about the person whose heart was keeping me alive. I got to know more about Danielle and her family. Charlotte said something only someone so close to the Lord could comprehend: "After getting to know you," she explained through tears of relief, "I now know that my daughter's purpose on earth was to be here so when you needed a new heart, she could give you hers."

How could a mom say something like that after losing her daughter? Danielle was a Christian, and she demonstrated it by her giving and loving lifestyle. And Danielle is still who she is, and I am who I am, but part of me has a piece of Danielle that God holds in high esteem—her heart. I cannot be who I am without Danielle's heart keeping me alive.

"But by the grace of God I am what I am . . ." This verse is clipped onto the bulletin board in my kitchen, reminding me quite often of who I am in God's eyes. No matter what I do wrong, whatever pain I suffer, whatever failures I despair over, I am exactly who God made me to be. And it was His plan that Danielle's life would become part of mine.

I now have an extended family that I am very connected to. Besides the physical connection, there is an emotional connection and a spiritual connection. All of us have gone through difficult situations to be where God wanted us to be, but embracing the plan and purpose for our lives allows all of us to continue on His path and to remain faithful in His care.

You are exactly who God intended you to be also. Time and experience may mold you and smooth out the rough edges, but He made no mistake when He created you.

8 Chapter 8
Time Keeps on Ticking

Fly Like an Eagle

Fly like an eagle, Let my spirit carry me
I want to fly like an eagle, Till I'm free
Oh, Lord, through the revolution

Time keeps on slippin', slippin', slippin'
Into the future
Time keeps on slippin', slippin', slippin'
Into the future ...

Steve Miller, "Fly Like an Eagle." The Steve Miller Band, Capitol, 1976

Time is something of an oddity. It's a word given much reverence in all of life. We sing about it, wonder about it, lose it, want it, and need more of it. Many are familiar with the lines from Ecclesiastes 3:1-8, "There is a time for everything . . ." King Solomon wrote this after he expounds on the concept of time: "Whatever is has already been, and what will be has been before; and God will call the past to account" (NIV). So what is the importance of time and why do we mull over the past, worry about the present, and anticipate and plan the future?

As I grew up in New York and learned to live in the craziness of its daily grind, I never had a chance to think about time. It was not an affordable commodity. You just knew a 15-mile trip in rush hour traffic would take 45 minutes. A trip to register your car at the Department of Motor Vehicles was a flat three to five hour wait—no slack given.

The express line at the grocery store was the longest line, so even though the amount of groceries per order was less, the time waiting was not. Emergencies were not shielded from the lack of time. If you had to visit the ER, you'd better be sure it wasn't life threatening!

New York City's motto "The City That Never Sleeps," is relative to its 24-hour subway system and constant drones of traffic and people. Living there is a blur and now that I live in a smaller city with rush hour traffic lasting possibly five to ten minutes, I have to say, time is more of a reality.

Why do we need more time? So we can fill it with things we must do, necessary restraints our lives impress on us. We think of time lost in the past and mourn it. "If only I had …" The past is a part of our lives, and the Lord does take into account what we do with our life here on earth, but "there is no time like the present." You and I can be responsible only for what happens today. We plan our futures the best we can, we work to make each day better than the one before, and we can only hope what we do brings the best result.

King Solomon contemplates how man works and plans and counts the minutes he wished he had, "So I saw that there is nothing better for a man than to enjoy his work, because that is his lot. For who can bring him to see what will happen after him?" (Ecclesiastes 3:22 NIV) His is a sobering look at time and its passing.

After moving away from New York, and being gone almost ten years, my husband and I returned for a visit. We forgot how treacherous it is to drive the speed limit even in the far right lane. I can't even tell you how many times we were forced to go faster or be escorted out of the lane we were in. It's just how New York and other large cities around the world operate.

A friend riding with us one day became impatient with my husband's driving. He was tormented that we took our time in the store, mulled about the shops we visited, and stopped to admire our surroundings. "You guys are no longer *engaged* in life!" was his outbreak. Honest and frustrated, I always consider his words.

Engaged in life? Engaged is associated with being busy, occupied, or involved in conflict. People who are engaged with life are sometimes engrossed with their days.

Now, consider those who are terminally ill, divorced, financially ruined, raising rebellious children, dealing with broken relationships, agonizing over unfulfilled promise, and torn dreams—how much time do they need to find peace? How much time is enough to drive them to their goal or desires?

I have learned to pass over the quantity of time in my own life. I don't worry anymore about being engaged in life. Instead I am determined to be absorbed with life, knowing how precious every chance is to work and live and be productive. "Behold, we count them happy which endure. Ye have heard of the patience of Job, and have seen the end of the LORD; that the LORD is very pitiful, and of tender mercy" (James 5:11 KJV).

I was working on a computer project at home one day for The King's *High* Way Ministries where I am employed, and something in the program would shut down each time I was ready to complete it. Just as I would be at the very end, the screen would blink—and it was gone! I was becoming frustrated when I realized I needed to take a breath and pray. I did. Then I rebooted the computer to give it a break. As I looked at the screen booting up and launched my program again, I anticipated another failure.

Suddenly, the Lord spoke loudly to me, "*You may be doing the work, but I am doing the miracle!*" It was loud and clear that I needed to rest and stop rushing the time.

Leaving my office, I walked outside to fill the bird feeders in my backyard. It was a cold, winter day and the crisp air cleared my head. The birds were so hungry, they filled the trees around me with chatter and anticipation. "*Time*," the Lord spoke to me, "*is not a concern of mine and should not be allowed to consume you. Use it wisely*."

A few days later, my Bible reading for the day was supposed to be Psalm 7, but something led me to read Psalm 30. There was no particular reason, I just felt like the Lord wanted me to read it. As usual, it was perfect timing. Psalm 30 is all about God's promises. And they were promises that I needed to hear.

> O LORD my God, I cried unto thee, and thou hast healed me. O LORD, thou hast brought up my soul from the grave: thou hast kept me alive, that I should not go down to the pit. Hear, O LORD, and have mercy upon me: LORD, be thou my helper. Thou hast turned for me my mourning into dancing: thou hast put off my sackcloth, and girded me with gladness (Psalm 30:2-3,10-11 KJV).

I questioned when these things would happen: healing, keep me alive, mercy, dancing, and gladness. Time has no meaning to God. If I could just grasp this fact and keep my thoughts from straying from the truth, I would not have to worry anymore about timing. We all have to remember this and try to eliminate time in our prayers and requests. Our future is the present to God.

Many of us have requests that we would like answered in a timeframe we can handle. For me, a new blockage could attack my coronary arteries. My friend Jeff, electrocuted years ago, no arms, and in a wheelchair, doesn't know how long he will live. How many countless people have jobs without security? There are many with family members away at war in foreign countries. The scenarios can go on endlessly if we all consider the way time makes itself an intrusion that demeans our faith. And we can easily lose faith as we seem to lose time.

A tragic story appeared on February 9, 2008, as a tiny headline from the Associated Press: "Bride dies during marriage's first dance."

> Kim Sjostrom wanted a real-life version of the film "My Big Fat Greek Wedding," which played in the background as friends fixed her hair and makeup before her own marriage ceremony.
>
> But less than an hour after she and Teddy Efkarpides were wed, Sjostrom crumpled in her husband's arms during a Greek song that means "Love Me."
>
> At 36, Sjostrom was dead from heart disease.
>
> Sjostrom carried blue and white flowers during the ceremony—the colors of the Greek flag—as she exchanged vows with Efkarpides, a 43-year-old carpenter and Navy veteran. They had met three years to the day before the Jan. 19 wedding.
>
> During the couple's first dance, Sjostrom complained of being lightheaded. Efkarpides thought his wife, a diabetic, needed sugar, but she collapsed.
>
> Wedding guests, paramedics and doctors at a nearby hospital were unable to revive her.
>
> He [Efkarpides] consoles himself by reading a list of "101 Reasons Why I Love You" that Sjostrom gave him their first Christmas together. "Number 1. You make me smile."
>
> No. 98 is especially difficult: "You're the one I want to grow old with."[53]

It's said that this couple never got to live out their lives as they planned. What might they have done differently if they had known their wedding day would be the last day they were together?

If all of us would consider the frailty of time, we would probably treat each other better. We would live our lives differently. The things that derail us would no longer have such a disastrous effect on our emotions and choices. We can't know the future—even the next few minutes of time. But we can live our lives like we do.

> Don't be so concerned about the future. *The future belongs to God.* He is in charge of all things and will take care of you completely. If you try to guess what is going to happen you will only worry yourself and anticipate trouble. *Live each day as it comes*. Francois de Fenelon, *The Seeking Heart.*[54]

A few months after my heart transplant, time moved on a slow, surrealistic course. I was no longer counting how many days I waited for a donor heart to become available. I was simply—counting. *It's been three weeks*, I considered, *and I am still at the hospital several days at a time for x-rays, blood work, biopsies of my heart, appointments . . . I thought going home from the hospital meant the beginning of my new existence, my new lease on life. Instead, it was a new world with new conditions*.

I remember my transplant nurse/coordinator telling me early on, "Don't let the doctors catch you using a wheelchair while you are here for testing. They want you to walk on your own." It's easy for a "normal" person to roll those words out. The transplant program included a rigorous schedule as soon as you got discharged. With all the testing needing to be done, you would find yourself walking from one end of the hospital to another, and many times traveling through outstretched hallways that seemingly never ended.

The constant routine was dragging me down and the assault on my body left me worn-out with a lot of time to think. I know I dwelled on my situation more then I should have, more than was healthy for me. But one thing that nagged at my disconcerted thoughts was, *Did I really need this heart transplant?* I am sure the four years of health care personnel doubting my condition contributed to my own doubts. I wanted to know for sure.

At my next appointment, after all day testing, I was ready to see the heart transplant surgeon. I went through the nurse intake, weigh-in, and medication check, and waited for the doctor to come in. After his assessment, and the usual small talk, I asked him if I could speak to him privately. "I have a question to ask you," I spoke softly as he looked into my eyes, searching for an indication of my state of mind.

We went into his back office. "Sit," he said.

"Oh no, that's okay. This will only take a moment." I was so nervous about asking him a question I thought might make him feel awkward. "Dr. Sandler, did I really need this heart transplant? I mean, so many times I was told things were in my mind. Would you and Dr. Icenogle have done this transplant if I hadn't needed it?"

His big, Russian brown eyes looked at me with soothing mercy and love. He grabbed me and gave me his characteristic bear hug. Holding me tight, he spoke calmly, "You're heart was a capital 'G'—'G' for garbage. I don't know how you lasted as long as you did and you would not have lasted much longer."

That was what I needed to hear. My doubting came to an end. This man had his hands in my chest. He held my heart, the heart I was born with, and cut it out to replace it with a new heart. Although this new heart had physical impairments, it would come to beat strongly and keep me alive for much longer than any of us could know.

I am reminded of this message of hope each time I hear my heart beat. At night, when it is really quiet and I am lying in bed, I can hear and feel this new heart beating in my chest. It reminds me of Ezekiel's message of hope to God's people. Ezekiel chose to always obey God, and sometimes the things God asked him to do were very dramatic and difficult. Still, Ezekiel continued to proclaim God's Word.

In Ezekiel 36:26, God promised to restore Israel not only physically but with a new spiritual heart:

> "Moreover, I will give you a new heart and put a new spirit within you; and I will remove the heart of stone from your flesh and give you a heart of flesh." (NASB)

"Stony" is an interesting way to describe their prior heart. When someone has had a lot of damage to their physical heart, the heart muscle becomes hard and unmovable. Webster's defines "stony" as "unfeeling; merciless, motionless or rigid, hardhearted and unfeeling, unemotional." We know Israel suffered all of these characteristics, but God had a better way for them to follow, a path to a new heart.

For me, getting a new heart not only gave me a new life physically, it also renewed me spiritually. I realize the miracle of my transplant and can now share the many ways God healed me, restored me, and grew me into who I am today. But the wait for this miracle was the most difficult wait I ever endured.

> Waiting is part of life, including life in the Spirit. . . . "Stay" is not a pleasant command. We want to get on with it. Waiting time feels like wasting time to us.

But notice where the waiting is located—between "what my Father has promised" and "being clothed with power from on high." We wait between the promise and the power, between believing God will do it and knowing He has done it, between the prayer and the praise, between what the Bible says and what the Spirit says.

This is the spiritual train depot, with its hard seats, gray walls, and stone floor. The waiting area is silent, cold, and nondescript—and there's nothing you can do about it. Ah—could this be the purpose of waiting? Between the power and the promise, God want us to stop "doing" and just "be" still, "be" patient, "be" faithful. In your attitude of stillness, patience, and faithfulness, God will open your life to receive the promise of the power.

If you are waiting today, remember: the promise is good the power will come.

Silently now I wait for Thee,
Ready, my God, Thy will to see.
Open my heart, illumine me,
Spirit divine.

Clara H. Scott ("Open My Eyes, That I May See")
Richard Parrott, *Come Ye Apart* (now called *Reflections*) is a quarterly devotional published by the Nazarene Publishing House

If you are willing to wait forever, chances are you won't have to wait long. At times throughout my illness, time and waiting were not even a choice. Time was an affliction that taunted me in a contemptuous way.

I waited often for doctor's appointments that were scheduled weeks or months away when I felt I needed to see someone sooner. I waited hours in the ER, with my husband propped up in a chair, leaning against the wall as he tried to rest his mind and body worn-out from the frequent heart attack scares. I watched the clock in my hospital room in anticipation of a transport employee coming with a stretcher to shuttle me to an operating room for a surgery or procedure.

How many days before I could go home, how many hours before I could see the doctor, how many weeks of chemo, how many days until I could receive a donor heart so I could stop counting how many days I may live. Time never let me stop wondering until I learned to stop counting.

Four months after receiving my heart transplant, I contracted a dangerous virus called CMV or cytomegalovirus. In most people, the virus will flare up a bit and then a healthy immune system will keep it at bay. But being immune compromised, so that my body would not reject my donor heart, the virus could become deadly as it spread throughout my bloodstream.

The only form of treatment to make this virus, a permanent resident in my system go dormant, is an antiviral IV medicine similar to chemotherapy. I was admitted to the hospital as soon as the CMV was discovered and started on an IV treatment of this chemotherapy two times a day—every day. The treatments made me sick, but were not near as bad as actual chemotherapy. When it was found that I could tolerate the chemotherapy, I was sent home on it for another month or so with nursing care.

I counted the six weeks on this regimen as a period of time that I could tolerate and then be rid of to continue on my road to recovery. When it was done, I celebrated as the tubing was removed from my arm.

A week or two later, the virus reared its ugly head again. Once more I was admitted and started on the chemo treatments. This time, stronger doses were administered in hopes of the virus staying dormant. But after the prescribed treatment at home, it returned once more. This time, testing was done to see if I was resistant to the medicine being used. I was. In fact, because the form of the virus I had (has 52 strains,) was resistant to the type of IV medication I was on, it meant it would not respond to any of the medicines in the same category. It was time to try another course of something more powerful.

The only option left was a very strong chemotherapy that had been used only one time in 20 years by my heart transplant team. It would mean having the treatments two times a day for 30 days and in the hospital only—not at home. The medicine would make me very sick, they told me. They were right!

Each treatment was preceded by an injection of Benadryl and a tranquilizer to prepare my body for the assault. As my heart surgeon put it, "It will be like having gasoline poured into your veins." The Benadryl was to help with the nausea and the tranquilizer was needed to help with the spasms and seizures caused by the chemotherapy. The treatments were done during the day and at night, so by the time I recovered from one, the next treatment was being started.

Although the hospital did its best to accommodate me, 30 days locked in an isolation room with limited walks in the hallways and unbearable side effects made for a long time to be incarcerated.

Time ticked steadily by on the large clock on the drab hospital room wall. Often I was too sick to care, but sometimes I would just lie on the bed, fighting the nausea and hoping for the last day to arrive. The days dragged on, meeting each other with the same routine and dread as the one before.

I thought about a lesson in endurance my mother-in-law Rose had taught me years before. I wanted to bake Christmas cookies with her and excitedly gathered all the ingredients and joined her in her kitchen. She offered plenty of skill and wisdom and we planned on baking the entire day.

One of the toppings I bought for the cookies were tiny, red cinnamon candies. After I arranged the ingredients on the kitchen table, I took the two-pound bag of them and tried to open it—carefully. But as I struggled to pull the plastic bag apart, it ripped, sending tiny round candies all over the linoleum floor.

"I'll get the broom," I lamented.

"Oh no!" insisted my mother-in-law. "You will get down on your hands and knees and pick up each one, carefully checking for dirt, and place them in this plastic bowl. When I was a little girl growing up in Brooklyn, my mother would buy a bag of lentils and we would have to sift through pounds of them and pick out all the little twigs and pebbles. Nothing was wasted or taken for granted. It taught all of us endurance and you are going to learn endurance now."

So I got down on the floor and started picking up each little red pearl, thinking of her story and lesson—a good lesson for me to learn. It took time to pick through each one and place them in the bowl, but when I was done, I was impressed with my small yet meaningful accomplishment. It was a lesson I will keep with me forever.

I endured day after day of treatment and when the chemotherapy was done after 30 grueling days, I was free to finally go home. I never wanted to go through that again and I knew it would take a while to recover from the side effects. I was discharged and the nurse called for a wheelchair to take me down to the entrance where John was waiting with the car.

"Oh, please let me walk down on my own," I begged the nurse. "I want to be as normal as possible." I took my bag and walked to the elevators. When I emerged out of the front doors of the hospital lobby, the fresh air was wonderful and I relished it all the way home, as the breeze from the car's open window blew on my face.

But shortly after my freedom was granted, the CMV virus came back once again. This was unheard of and my doctors searched for anything else they could do before they once again would have to imprison me to another bout of chemotherapy. They were not sure how much more my kidneys and body could take, and they were not sure how much I could take.

After much deliberation, I was again admitted for another month of torture. As I did before, I crossed off the days on the calendar hanging from my bulletin board. Once again, cards from friends and family decorated the room and my belongings took their place in the bedside dresser. Healthy snacks protruded from the top drawer and I stared at the dark TV screen, uninterested in its dribble of noise and irritating shows.

I kept busy, drawing with colored markers on the white poster board tacked to the wall that my friend Terry brought for me. I read when I was able, worked on my computer when I could focus, and once again lamented for the end to come. Time? There was lots of it, but I was trapped in a pallid time warp as, again, one day melded into another.

"God is extremely diligent and painfully slow," Chuck Swindoll touted. His words were so profound when I heard them. God will always complete what He needs to in our lives, but He will take as long as He needs to accomplish this completion of His will for us.

Like the words of Richard Parrott, in his devotional in *Come Ye Apart*, *stay* is not a fun word.

> I am going to send you what my Father has promised; but stay in the city until you have been clothed with power from on high (Luke 24:49 NIV).

"Stay until you have been clothed with power from on high." If only we could all learn to stay and wait patiently, time would no longer be an enemy and the future would not have to be a fearful unknown. The chemotherapy lasted another month and then I had to go home and stay on it for an additional six months! The news was more than I could bear. Six months of daily treatments. I was reduced to one a day, but even cancer patients don't usually have chemotherapy every day for such a prolonged period of time.

By the time I finished the second round and went home to endure the additional six months, I had lost most of my hair, experienced terrible stomach problems, and felt like I was being poisoned. But I wanted to be "clothed with the power on high" God had promised. So I determined to beat the poison and kept my self focused on God's will for my life. I did as much as was physically possible at home, and sometimes got a ride to the ministry office where I worked, toting my chemotherapy in a backpack, hooking up the bag of medicine, and hanging it on the door jamb in my office.

And I didn't stop living. Terry and I packed up the car one day and took the five-hour drive to Seattle to spend the day shopping and getting my mind off the torturous treatments. I hung the IV bottle from the visor in the front of the car and off we went. It was great to get out, and humorous to see the look on the teenager's face as she handed me my drink at the drive-thru while the IV dripped into my arm.

While life can be full of painful times and difficult circumstances, God equips all of us to endure it with flair and get through the tough times unscathed. It is our choice. A quote by an anonymous writer illustrates the benefit of painful endurance: "Pain is weakness leaving the body." And often the very pain that we fight to relieve ourselves of is the catalyst to make us stronger.

It took me a year to recover from the effects of this poisonous chemotherapy. And when I thought I was finally on the mend, another tragic accident put me back on the wheel of time. I broke my right leg in two places. It was bad enough that if I moved the bone the wrong way it would have required surgery.

John and I had gone to a family wedding in Florida and I was well enough to dance and enjoy the reception with friends and family. But on the last night of our trip, a very wonderful night in which we enjoyed fresh seafood for dinner and a walk on the ocean, I decided to bring some coconuts home to give out at the ministry. With an arm full of them, I stepped off the curb and jammed my foot between the sidewalk and parking space barrier. I never even hit the ground, but jammed my knee so badly, it fractured the tibia plateau on both the left and right side just under my knee.

It's strange how such a split second event can be remembered in slow motion. I knew as I went down that I had broken my leg, and the first thing I thought was *Oh poor John*, knowing he would have to take care of me once more. I also thought of the time I would have to be in a cast or wheelchair before I healed. It took 12 weeks with no ability to walk on or use my right leg. More counting. More waiting for a chance to be free. Time kept on ticking . . .

My leg is now healed, the chemotherapy is done, I am alive, and although time continues to propel me into the future, it is the present that really matters. God will take care of the time He dominates. Stay—until you have been clothed with power from on high.

Conclusion
What Is Your *Heart* Disease?

What is your heart disease? Marriage? Finances? Children that have gone astray? What do you choose to do with your situation? I cannot forget how I sunk to my knees when the Lord made clear what He was trying to say to Job: "Beware of turning to *evil*, which you seem to prefer to affliction" (36:21b). Beware of turning to *evil*—oh, those words struck me with powerful conviction. When afflicted with the pain of tragedy in life, it is easy to choose evil. Evil could be anger, bitterness, vengefulness, or the other side of the spectrum—apathy, lack of emotion or that numb lethargy that comes with shock. All these things are ways to avoid facing affliction head-on.

I found out very quickly that avoiding the affliction I had grown weary of caused me to choose evil. My moods and emotions became a whirlwind running out of control. But when I faced the pressure head-on and put my trust in the Lord, forging ahead to combat the pain, the result was empowering. If I was joyful in the face of affliction, people around me saw the power of God. They could see the strength was not mine but supernatural. God is given the glory. He is certainly made strong in our weakness.

> But he said to me, "My grace is sufficient for you, for my power is made perfect in weakness." Therefore I will boast all the more gladly about my weaknesses,

> so that Christ's power may rest on me. That is why, for Christ's sake, I delight in weaknesses, in insults, in hardships, in persecutions, in difficulties. *For when I am weak, then I am strong* (2 Corinthians 12:9,10 NIV, emphasis added).

Often it seems the things we treasure most in our lives are what is taken away from us. Loss does much for breaking our hearts and our faith. The darkness of the enemy, as we know him, is supreme at hiding our treasures under his terror. But God never takes away what we treasure here on earth without revealing more treasure gained by the very loss of the precious things we cleave to:

> I will go before you and make the rough places smooth; I will shatter the doors of bronze and cut through their iron bars. I will give you the treasures of darkness and hidden wealth of secret places, so that you may know that it is I, The LORD, the God of Israel, who calls you by your name (Isaiah 45:2,3 NASB).

Chuck Swindoll, in his Bible study guide *Hope in Hurtful Times*, lists three reasons for suffering:

> That we might be prepared to comfort others.
> That we might not trust in ourselves.
> That we might learn to give thanks in everything.

Jonah, an Old Testament writer, experienced these three concepts first hand. After disobeying God, he was swallowed up by a great fish, vomited out on shore after three days in its belly and then, after he completes his task in Nineveh, faces yet more despairing times:

> Then the LORD God provided a vine and made it grow up over Jonah to give shade for his head to ease his discomfort, and Jonah was very happy about the vine. But at dawn the next day God provided a worm, which chewed the vine so that it withered. When the sun rose, God provided a scorching east wind, and the sun blazed on Jonah's head so that he grew faint. He wanted to die, and said, "It would be better for me to die than to live." But God said to Jonah, "Do you have a right to be angry about the vine?" "I do," he said. "I am angry enough to die." But the LORD said, "You have been concerned about this vine, though you did not tend it or make it grow. It sprang up overnight and died overnight. But Nineveh has more than a hundred and twenty thousand people who cannot tell their right hand from their left, and many cattle as well. Should I not be concerned about that great city?" (Jonah 4:6-11 NIV)

Jonah was self-absorbed. Instead of seeking the Lord for his strength, he looked to himself and found only anger. God tried to get his attention by allowing the vine to wither up. This was a small inconvenience compared to the needs of the people in Nineveh. God's grace was there to sustain him, but he chose not to accept it.

The apostle Paul wrote much about pain, suffering, and heartache. But in all his writings, his drive is always towards grace. Swindoll explains Paul's salutation found in 2 Corinthians 1:2:

> Grace is . . . God doing for us that which we don't deserve and cannot repay. And in its wake comes peace. Grace and peace don't come from ourselves—no matter

> how positive our thoughts; or from others—no matter how assuring their counsel. They come only from God.[55]

Everyday difficulties and personal hardships and pain can lead us to choose one of two paths. Either we allow these tremors to give birth to contaminating seeds of embitterment or we allow God to be the strength of our hearts and our portion forever.

Mike Webb of Mission Romania, a ministry based in Sierra Vista, Arizona, wrote:

> It seems that there is in our hearts some little, locked, dark room full of foul, corrupting stuff that God means to get at and take care of. These areas are like little imps which enslave us and we are deceived into thinking we NEED them. Recognizing these "imps" is not enough for healing. There must be a decision of the will to tie them to the altar of God and let HIM destroy them with holy fire. Thus, our own private cremation.[56]

I recall a conversation I had with a friend's daughter as we ate lunch together. Misty, just 18 years old, had suffered for years from an unknown illness. Plagued with weakness, headaches, stomach troubles, and other symptoms, she had become angry and bitter. Her hopelessness was evident by her expression of defeat.

"It's like I'm in the hurling of a hurricane. When will I get to the eye of the storm? I know there will be calm and rest there."

My reply had to be realistic, "It's actually a tornado! And the storm will not end until we reach heaven." Her look was disheartened and frustrated as she listened with disregard. I was trying to encourage her from my seasoned understanding of the will God has for each of our lives. He knows when we can be effective as Christians, and finding His will for our lives frees us to forge ahead without despair.

I know I can't keep looking back. The driving force in my life is to look ahead.

> Brethren, I do not count myself to have apprehended; but one thing I do, forgetting those things which are behind and reaching forward to those things which are ahead, I press toward the goal for the prize of the upward call of God in Christ Jesus (Philippians 3: 13,14 NKJV).

John was by my side when the first open heart surgery almost took my life. The doctor called in the chaplain and prepared John for me to die. But I made it—again and again. My cardiologist told me more than once I am the worst patient he has ever encountered. One new doctor was real quiet after sitting with me for two hours. She apologized and said she was not usually so quiet but she was dumbfounded at all I survived. Another doctor I saw—world famous—couldn't believe I was still alive.

At times, the news was not good. Once when I asked my cardiologist, Dr. Canaday, about my main artery, he said he had cleaned it out and worked on it way more times than recommended. As he put it, "We have gone where no man has gone before." The wall of the artery became very thin and could collapse at any time if he had to clean it out again.

Each day I woke up not knowing if it would be the day my artery blocks up once again. My arteries would block up 99 percent within a week where it would take a year or more for someone else. I had much cause to worry—constantly. It took me a long time to actually get to a point where worry was a far-off threat that I could anticipate and stop before it became a problem.

One Sunday at church, the youth pastor shared his teaching on worry based on Matthew 6:25-34. He asked the congregation a question: "Who here knows the secret to not worrying? If you do, please see me after the service."

I wanted to raise my hand with the answer when he asked his question. I don't think he expected anyone to approach him but if church hadn't been so crowded, I would have spoken to him after the service. I wanted to let him know I had reached a point where worry was only a distant fraction of my days. With all I survived and had been through, how could I worry when God is always taking care of the things that could harm me? It was the same message of hope the prophet Jeremiah carried to the remnant exiled from Jerusalem to Babylon by Nebuchadnezzar: " 'For I know the plans I have for you,' declares the LORD, 'plans to prosper you and not to harm you, plans to give you hope and a future' " (Jeremiah 29:11 NIV). We, too, can stand on the same promise today. Yet fear and worry seem to be bred into us from our childhood.

When I was a small girl, I was terrified of thunderstorms, especially when they came during the night. The home I grew up in was a three-level split and the bedrooms upstairs always stayed hot after a long, summer day.

Being that I grew up with 12 siblings, the master bedroom was used as a dormitory with four of us sleeping together. There were windows on both sides of the room and when violent summer thunderstorms hit, the open screens exaggerated their fury. Although we were all together, those storms turned our crowded room into a lonely, scary place. A big oak tree's branches scraped against the house creating shrilly screeches while its leaves cast eerie shadows on the walls. I could smell the rain in the gentle breeze coming through windows and hear the distant thunder approaching.

In anticipation of the arrival of the storm, I would pull my blanket over my head, leaving a thin slit over my eyes so I could keep watch for lightning. I would imagine horrible destruction from lightning strikes or the oak tree coming down on the roof. I always feared the silent darkness of a power outage.

How I trembled under that quilt, my body becoming drenched with sweat. I would not dare to emerge from the protection of my cocoon until I was sure the storm had moved past. Then when I knew I was safe, I would throw the covers off and the cool, fresh air, sweetened from the rain, would breathe relief on my entire body. I was finally safe.

Worry is the storm we need not fear. It is the heavy, moist air trapped under the blanket of concern.

With all I have been through, worry can no longer entrap me. I am thankful to be alive. Yes, I am. I am thankful I am not living in Iraq because I would be dead. I am thankful my husband is a man of God and has stuck by me in all the lonely and painful hours. I am thankful I can walk and drive and get around. There are so many things to be thankful for. But if I look at the list, none of them are eternal.

> But all of you who held fast to the LORD your God are still alive today (Deuteronomy 4:4 NIV).

After all I have been through and will continue to go through, the one thing I meditate on each day is being thankful for my faith in a God who is bigger than any trial I will face. Many times I have had people offer suggestions of why I am sick and have not been healed. I don't pray with an agenda and I hardly pray for healing anymore. Instead, I pray I will be faithful and worthy to be a witness of the power of God. This is much bigger than healing.

I had a friend say, "If you had cancer, you'd either be better by now or dead." So how do I continue to endure and still give thanks? I hold onto the Word of God, I pray always and I surrender everything to God. Remember what the Lord spoke to me earlier? "I cannot heal you until you are ready to accept how I choose to heal you—and I am not finished yet." So I must surrender all I am to Him and trust Him. And remember the anchors God gave me to hold on in the storms?

> Beware of turning to evil, which you seem to prefer to affliction (Job 36:21 NIV).

> Do not grieve, for the joy of the LORD is your strength (Nehemiah 8:10b NIV).

> Deal courageously, and the LORD shall be with the good (2 Chronicles 19:11b KJV).

Nancy DeMoss writes this about thankfulness:

> Last Thanksgiving, I got a letter from a dear 89-year-old couple, Del Fehsenfeld, Sr. and his wife Dot. I call them Grandma and Grandpa Fehsenfeld. This is a thankful couple. And here is the letter they sent out as a thanksgiving letter to their friends. They said:

> "My dear friends and co-workers in Christ,

> In Christ, we have everything we need and want. Although Mrs. Fehsenfeld and I have been frequenting the doctor more than we would prefer" (and that's an understatement, by the way. They both had some real serious health challenges in the last year.)

They go on to say, "We are still glad and rejoice that He has been our sufficiency through aches, pains and operations. We ask you to join us in obeying His command, 'In everything give thanks; for this is the will of God in Christ Jesus for you, 1 Thessalonians 5:18.' "

What a challenge to me in my mid-40s whining and complaining about the little things in life that throw me off to hear this couple approaching 90 saying, "We're thankful."

Sometimes it's really hard to give thanks. Sometimes it's costly to give thanks. Sometimes you have to offer a sacrifice of thanksgiving—through your tears—to say, "Lord, though I do not understand why You would have me go through these circumstances, though I do not understand why I am receiving these divorce papers that I don't want, I don't understand why my son or daughter is responding in these ways that are not pleasing to You, I choose in the midst of a struggle, in the midst of the pressure, in the midst of the problems, I choose to give You thanks because You are still God. And You are still good and You are accomplishing Your purposes through every circumstance that is in my life."[57]

How often now I consider my life here on earth as each day brings me one more opportunity to make a difference. Maybe something I do or say can bring encouragement to someone else in a heart-wrenching situation. I deal with a physically broken heart, but that does not mean I do not also deal with emotional and spiritual brokenness. My dreadful medical problems may have physically damaged my heart that carries the life-blood through my body, but the soul God made in me resides in my spiritual heart. It is in this spiritual heart that I really carry the life God is interested in.

> Right now, you may be going through the hardest time you've ever faced. Your life may be unsettled, and things may look hopeless. Could it be a lost job? Maybe your financial situation is out of control. There seems to be no way out for you. Every avenue you turn to fills you with more stress, confusion and weariness.
>
> That is when the mind begins to reason, "How can I have peace with all of this debt hanging over my head? How can I possibly be calm when I need a financial miracle? I'm at the end of my rope. The future seems so uncertain."
>
> Maybe your family is in a crisis, or your marriage is struggling, or your health is failing, and there seems to be no hope ahead. You tell yourself, "If I could just see some light at the end of the tunnel. Yet all I see is uncertainty on all sides. If I could just get healing for my body — get deliverance for my child — get out of debt — then I'd have peace. Give me a miracle, and I'll know peace."
>
> When Christ promised the disciples his peace, it was as if he was saying to them (as well as to us today): "I know you don't understand the hard times that you face. You don't comprehend the Cross and the suffering I am about to face. Yes, you are about to be tried beyond

your human capacity to endure. You're going to be confused and feel forsaken by the Father."

It doesn't matter what you're going through. Your life may look like it has been struck by a tornado. You may endure trials that cause others to look at you as a modern-day Job. But in the midst of your troubles, when you call on the Holy Spirit to baptize you in the peace of Christ, he will do it.

People will point to you and say, "That person's world has come completely apart. Yet he's determined to trust God's Word, live or die. How can he do it? How does he go on? He should have quit long ago. Yet he hasn't given up. And through it all, he hasn't compromised anything he believes. What amazing peace! It's beyond understanding. "The Importance of Having the Peace of Christ." David Wilkerson[58]

This book really has no ending. My life, as many days as I have left here on earth, will continue regardless of how much I learn or how much closer I grow to the Lord. The tornado of trials will remain, hurling around me, and the same power that allows turmoil and tribulation in my life will carry me closer and closer to heaven.

My physical heart was failing until I received new life from Danielle—my angel on earth. More essential is the health of my spiritual heart which received new life through Christ.

A heart like mine must find God's will for my life and your heart must also navigate the path and process to bring you to His will and purpose for your own life.

Glossary*

*The following are terms used in the world of cardiology and in other similar medical fields. I have prepared this glossary to be as *accurate as possible*, but have modified some of the definitions to relate to the layman in all of us. DO NOT use this glossary for a medical diagnosis or as a replacement for a proper assessment by a medical doctor. This information is provided for reference only.

A

ablation – Ablation is used to treat abnormal heart rhythms. Nonsurgical ablation, used for many types of arrhythmias, is performed in a special lab called the electrophysiology (EP) laboratory. During this non-surgical procedure a catheter is inserted into a specific area of the heart. A special machine directs energy through the catheter to small areas of the heart muscle that causes the abnormal heart rhythm. This energy "disconnects" the pathway of the abnormal rhythm. It can also be used to disconnect the electrical pathway between the upper chambers and the lower chambers of the heart. In addition to re-establishing a normal heart rhythm in people with certain arrhythmias, ablation therapy can help control the heart rate in people with rapid arrhythmias, and reduce the risk of blood clots and strokes. (WebMD.com)

abnormal heart rhythm – see **arrhythmia**

acute coronary artery disease – Acute coronary artery disease is chest pain and other symptoms that happen because the heart does not get enough blood. It includes unstable angina and heart attack. Acute coronary syndrome happens because plaque narrows or blocks the arteries that supply blood to the heart. Plaque is made of cholesterol and other things. Over time, plaque can build up in the arteries. This is known as coronary artery disease. <WebMD.com>

adrenaline (epinephrine) – One of the body's many hormones is adrenaline. Higher amounts of the hormone epinephrine (adrenaline) in blood in early morning can cause heart attacks.

angiogenesis – Angiogenesis is a natural process in the body that involves the growth of new blood vessels. It can occur during coronary artery disease, peripheral artery disease and stroke when there's insufficient blood supply and oxygen to the tissues, a condition known as ischemia. The body's first response to less blood flow to the heart is to grow tiny new "collateral" vessels to help blood flow around the blockage. For unknown reasons, the process eventually switches off. Some proteins in the body can help trigger new blood vessel growth and so increase the oxygen supply to the ischemic tissue. Such angiogenic proteins include the vascular endothelial growth factor (VEGF) and fibroblast growth factor (FGF). (American Heart Association)

AMA – "Against Medical Advice" meaning a patient has made a decision that is deemed medically unsound by the physician such as signing yourself out of the hospital before recommendation.

angiogram – see **catheterization**

angioplasty – A procedure in which the narrowing in the wall of a blood vessel is treated by inflating a balloon attached to the tip of a catheter and running it up through an artery with a catheter wire.

arrhythmia – An irregular heartbeat is an arrhythmia (also called dysrhythmia). Heart rates can also be irregular. A normal heart rate is 50 to 100 beats per minute. Arrhythmias and abnormal heart rates don't necessarily occur together. Arrhythmias can occur with a normal heart rate or with heart rates that are slow (called bradyarrhythmias—less than 60 beats per minute). Arrhythmias can also occur with rapid heart rates (called tachyarrhythmias—faster than 100 beats per minute). <WebMD.com>

B

ballooning – With simple angioplasty, a balloon at the end of a long tube is threaded through an artery in the groin. The doctor guides the tube up the artery and into the heart, inflating the balloon where the vessel has narrowed. The balloon opens up the walls of the vessel. Then it is deflated and removed. (WebMD.com)

blockage – If there is too much cholesterol in the bloodstream, the excess may be deposited in arteries, including the coronary (heart) arteries, where it contributes to the narrowing and blockages that cause the signs and symptoms of heart disease. <WebMD.com>

blood pressure – The force exerted by the blood upon the walls of the arteries. The pressure in the arteries originates in the pumping action of the heart, and pressure waves can be felt at the wrist and at other points where arteries lie near the surface of the body. Because the heart can pump blood into the large arteries more quickly than it can be absorbed and released by the tiny arterioles and capillaries, considerable inner pressure always exists in the arteries. The contraction of the heart (systole) causes the blood pressure to rise to its highest point, and relaxation of the heart (diastole) brings the pressure down to its lowest point. (Columbia University Press Encyclopedia)

blood transfusion – The transfer of blood from one person to another. Transfusions are performed to replace a substantial loss of blood and as supportive treatment in certain diseases and blood disorders. (Columbia University Press Encyclopedia)

bone density – Bone density tests (also called bone mineral density tests or bone scans) evaluate the strength of your bones by measuring a small part of one or a few bones. Knowing the strength of your bones can help your doctor recommend prevention steps and osteoporosis medication, if needed, to prevent bone loss and fractures. <WebMD.com>

brachytherapy – Placing stents in arteries during angioplasty is very effective at keeping heart blood vessels open. But even when stents are implanted, arteries narrow again in up to 20% of people. This renarrowing is called in-stent restenosis. Most restenosis is due to scar tissue that forms in response to the injury created when the stent was implanted. Some scar tissue is useful as it covers the metal stent and helps prevent blood clots from forming. In some people, however, the process does not stop, and the scar tissue recloses the artery. When restenosis occurs, doctors can fix the problem by radiating the site of renarrowing. This is called brachytherapy. <WebMD.com>

bpm – Beats per minute; used to define heart rate.

bypass surgery – During coronary artery bypass graft surgery (also called CABG, or "cabbage") a blood vessel is removed or redirected from one area of the body and placed around the area or areas of narrowing to "bypass" the blockages and restore blood flow to the heart muscle. This vessel is called a graft. These substitute blood vessels can come from your chest, legs, or arms. They're safe to use because there are other pathways that take blood to and from those tissues. The surgeon will decide which graft(s) to use depending on the location of your blockage, the amount of blockage, and the size of your coronary arteries.

C

cardiologist – A specialized doctor who treats conditions related to the heart.

cardiopulmonary arrest – see **heart attack**

cartilage – A tough, elastic, fibrous connective tissue found in various parts of the body, such as the joints.

catheter – A flexible or rigid hollow tube employed to drain fluids from body cavities or to distend body passages.

catheterization – Cardiac catheterization (also called heart catheterization or coronary angiogram) is an invasive imaging procedure that allows your doctor to "see" how well your heart is functioning. During the test, a long, narrow tube, called a catheter, is inserted into a blood vessel in your arm or leg and guided to your heart with the aid of a special X-ray machine. Contrast dye is injected through the catheter so that X-ray movies of your valves, coronary arteries, and heart chambers can be created. (WebMD.com)

catheterization wire – To perform a heart catheterization, a thin, flexible tube called a catheter (or wire) is threaded through a blood vessel in the groin, or sometimes in another location, and into the heart. Through the catheter, the doctor can measure pressures, take blood samples, and inject a special dye (contrast material) into the chambers of the heart or the coronary arteries. The doctor watches the movement of the dye through the heart's chambers and blood vessels. (WebMD.com)

centrifugal machine – A blood centrifuge utilizes the manageable force of gravity to separate the components of blood by spinning it at a high speed.

chemotherapy – Chemotherapy is the general term for any treatment involving the use of chemical agents to stop cancer cells from growing. Chemotherapy is designed to kill cancer cells. It can be administered through a vein, injected into a body cavity, or delivered orally in the form of a pill, depending on which drug is used.

clinical trial – In health care, clinical trials are conducted to allow safety and efficacy data to be collected for new drugs or devices. These can take place only when satisfactory information has been gathered on the quality of the product and its nonclinical safety. Depending on the type of product and the stage of its development, clinical trials initially enroll healthy volunteers and/or patients into small studies, followed by larger scale studies in patients that often compare the new product with the currently prescribed treatment. As positive safety data are gathered, the number of patients can be increased. The FDA (Food and Drug Administration) determines if a new product is safe and either approves or disproves it for manufacturing.

code blue – Often the term "code" is used as slang for a cardiopulmonary arrest happening to a patient in a hospital or clinic, requiring a team of providers (sometimes called a "code team") to rush to the specific location and begin immediate resuscitative efforts. Every hospital or clinic has its own system for disseminating information about emergencies, and many use the term "code" plus a color or number to signify exactly what kind of emergency is occurring. "Code Blue" is often used to refer to a cardiopulmonary arrest.

coding – Going into **cardiopulmonary arrest**

congenital – Of or pertaining to a condition present at birth, whether inherited or caused by the environment, esp. the uterine environment. (Dictionary.com)

coronary – Encircling in the manner of a crown; in cardiology this refers to the arteries of the heart and, by extension, to related diseases, defects or malfunctions of the heart.

coronary artery - Coronary arteries supply blood to the heart muscle. Like all other tissues in the body, the heart muscle needs oxygen-rich blood to function, and oxygen-depleted blood must be carried away. The coronary arteries consist of two main arteries: the right and left coronary arteries, and their two branches, the circumflex artery and the left anterior descending artery.

coronary spasms – Plaque is not always the cause of a heart attack. In rare cases, the coronary artery spasms and contracts, obstructing blood flow and causing chest pain. If severe, the spasm can completely block blood flow and cause a heart attack. Most of the time in these cases, atherosclerosis is also involved, although sometimes the arteries are clear. Cold weather, emotional stress, and other factors can cause these spasms. But in many other cases, it is not known what triggers them. These spasms cause angina, chest pain, and discomfort. (WebMD.com)

coronary vessel – Coronary circulation is the circulation of blood in the blood vessels that supply blood to and from the heart muscle itself. Although blood fills the chambers of the heart, the muscle tissue of the heart, or myocardium, is so thick that it requires coronary blood vessels to deliver blood deep into it. The vessels that deliver oxygen-rich blood to the myocardium are known as coronary arteries. (WebMD.com)

CT scan – Computed tomography, commonly known as a CT scan, combines multiple X-ray images with the aid of a computer to produce cross-sectional views of the body. Cardiac CT is a heart-imaging test that uses CT technology with or without intravenous (IV) contrast (dye) to visualize the heart anatomy, coronary circulation, and great vessels (which includes the aorta, pulmonary veins, and arteries). (WebMD.com)

CMV – Cytomegalovirus, or CMV, is found universally throughout all geographic locations and socioeconomic groups, and infects between 50% and 85% of adults in the United States by 40 years of age. Once a person becomes infected, the virus remains alive, but usually dormant within that person's body for life. Recurrent disease rarely occurs unless the person's immune system is suppressed due to therapeutic drugs or disease. Therefore, for the vast majority of people, CMV infection is not a serious problem. However, CMV infection is important to certain high-risk groups such as the risk of infection to the immune compromised person, such as organ transplant recipients and persons infected with human immunodeficiency virus (HIV). Infection with CMV is a major cause of disease and death in immune compromised patients, including organ transplant recipients, patients with cancer, patients receiving immunosuppressive drugs, and HIV-infected patients.

D

depression – Depression is a serious medical illness that involves the brain. It's more than just a feeling of being “down in the dumps” or “blue” for a few days. For the more than 20 million people in the United States who have depression, the feelings do not go away. They persist and interfere with everyday life. Symptoms can include sadness, loss of interest or pleasure in activities one used to enjoy, change in weight, difficulty sleeping or oversleeping, energy loss, feelings of worthlessness, thoughts of death or suicide. (http://www.nlm.nih.gov/medlineplus/depression.html)

diagonal artery – smaller branch of the coronary artery.

double bypass surgery – Coronary artery bypass surgery, also coronary arterybypass graft surgery, and colloquially heart bypass or bypass surgery is a surgical procedure performed to relieve angina and reduce the risk of death from coronary artery disease. The terms single bypass, double bypass, triple bypass, quadruple bypass, and quintuple bypass refer to the number of coronary arteries bypassed in the procedure. In other words, a double bypass means two coronary arteries are bypassed.

E

EKG/ECG – An electrocardiogram (EKG or ECG) is a test that checks for problems with the electrical activity of your heart. An EKG translates the heart's electrical activity into line tracings on paper. The spikes and dips in the line tracings are called waves. <WebMD.com>

electrical pathways – Flow of electricity within the heart: The heart's electrical system causes the heart to beat, controls the heart rate (the number of beats per minute), and has special pathways (conduction pathways) that carry the electrical signals throughout the lower heart chambers (ventricles) for each heartbeat. The electrical chain reaction that occurs in the heart is much like ripples on the calm surface of a pond.

electromagnetic field – The field of force associated with electric charge in motion, having both electric and magnetic components and containing a definite amount of electromagnetic energy. Magnetic fields can interrupt the proper functioning of a pacemaker.

electrophysiological cardiologist – These physicians have special training in the diagnosis and treatment of cardiac rhythm abnormalities. Electrophysiology is the study of cardiac arrhythmias, or abnormal heart rhythms.

electrophysiology – Diagnosing heart disease: electrophysiology testing - An electrophysiology (EP) study is a test that records the electrical activity and the electrical pathways of the heart. This test is used to help determine the cause of heart rhythm disturbances.

elevated pressure – Because blood is carried from the heart to all of your body's tissue and organs in vessels called arteries, blood pressure is the force of the blood pushing against the walls of those arteries. In fact, each time the heart beats (about 60-70 times a minute at rest), it pumps out blood into the arteries. Your blood pressure is at its greatest when the heart contracts and is pumping the blood. This is called systolic pressure. When the heart is at rest, in between beats, your blood pressure falls. This is the diastolic pressure. Blood pressure is always given as these two numbers, systolic and diastolic pressures. Both are important. Usually they are written one above or before the other, such as 120/80 mm Hg, with the top number the systolic and the bottom the diastolic. Different actions make your blood pressure go up or down. For example, if you run for a bus, your blood pressure goes up. When you sleep at night, your blood pressure goes down. These changes in blood pressure are normal. Some people have blood pressure that stays up all or most of the time. Their blood pushes against the walls of their arteries with higher-than-normal force. If untreated, this can lead to serious medical problems. <WebMD.com>

epinephrine – Epinephrine (see adrenaline) is a hormone.

F

femur artery – A large artery that starts in the lower abdomen and goes down into the thigh. It is the main artery of the thigh, supplying blood to the groin and lower extremities.

FGF-1 – Fibroblast growth factors, or FGFs, are a family of growth factors involved in angiogenesis, wound healing, and embryonic development.

full metal jacket – In terms of coronary arteries of the heart this means that metal stents have been placed in the entire artery, lining it completely.

H

heart attack – A heart attack occurs when blood flow to the heart is blocked. Without blood and the oxygen it carries, part of the heart starts to die. It's also called a myocardial infarction, or MI. Heart attacks happen when blood flow to the heart is blocked. This usually occurs because fatty deposits called plaque have built up inside the coronary arteries which supply blood to the heart. If a plaque breaks open, the body tries to fix it by forming a clot around it. Some heart attacks are sudden but most heart attacks start slowly, with mild pain or discomfort.

heart catheterization – see catheterization

hostel – An inexpensive, supervised lodging place for young people on bicycle trips, hikes, educational trips, etc.

HRV – Heart rate variability (HRV) refers to the beat-to-beat alterations in heart rate.

I

intervention – Also known as angioplasty or percutaneous coronary intervention

IV – An intravenous (inside the vein) device for delivering electrolyte solutions, medicines, and nutrients.

immune system – In simplest terms, the immune system is a balanced network of cells and organs that work together to defend you against disease. It blocks foreign proteins from getting into your body. If a few happen to sneak by your biological sentry, not to worry. With a powerful "search and destroy" task force, your body deploys a host of additional immune cell forces designed to hunt down these unwanted invaders and ultimately works to destroy them. <WebMD.com>

immune compromised – A state in which the immune system's ability to fight infectious disease is compromised or entirely absent. Most cases of immunodeficiency are acquired ("secondary") but some people are born with defects in the immune system, or primary immunodeficiency. Transplant patients take medications to suppress their immune system as an anti-rejection measure. A person who has an immunodeficiency of any kind is said to be immunocompromised. An immunocompromised person may be particularly vulnerable to opportunistic infections, in addition to normal infections that could affect everyone.

L

left anterior descending artery – The left anterior descending artery branches off the left coronary artery and supplies blood to the front of the heart.

lethargic – Sluggish, drowsy, tired.

Lou Gehrig's Disease – Lou Gehrig's disease, is a progressive wasting away of certain nerve cells of the brain and spinal column called motor neurons. The motor neurons control the voluntary muscles, which are the muscles that allow movement. ALS is a progressive, disabling, fatal disease. The course of the disease is different for everyone and some people live with ALS for many years. Walking, speaking, eating, swallowing, breathing, and other basic functions become more difficult with time. These problems can lead to injury, illness, and other complications. <WebMD.com>

N

Nitroglycerin – “Nitro” Nitroglycerin is a vasodilator, a medicine that opens blood vessels to improve blood flow. It is used to treat angina, a type of chest pain, that happens when there is not enough blood flowing to the heart. To improve blood flow to the heart, nitroglycerin opens up (dilates) the arteries in the heart (coronary arteries), which improves symptoms and reduces how hard the heart has to work.

NPO – “Nothing by Mouth” commonly used in the hospital meaning no food or drink allowed.

nuclear stress test – A stress test can be used to test for heart disease. Stress tests are tests performed by a doctor and/or trained technician to determine the amount of stress that your heart can manage before developing either an abnormal rhythm or evidence of ischemia (not enough blood flow to the heart muscle). The most commonly performed stress test is the *ex*ercise stress test—also called a stress test, exercise electrocardiogram, treadmill test, graded exercise test or stress ECG. This is a test used to provide information about how the heart responds to exertion. It usually involves walking on a treadmill or pedaling a stationary bike at increasing levels of difficulty, while your electrocardiogram, heart rate and blood pressure are monitored.

The *nuclear stress test*: This test helps to determine which parts of the heart are healthy and function normally and which are not. A very small and harmless amount of radioactive substance is injected into the patient, then the doctor uses a special camera to identify the rays emitted from the substance within the body. This produces clear pictures of the heart tissue on a monitor. These pictures are done both at rest and after exercise. Using this technique, a less than normal amount of thallium will be seen in those areas of the heart that have a decreased blood supply. <WebMD.com>

O

occlusion – A coronary occlusion is the partial or complete obstruction of blood flow in a coronary artery. This condition may cause a heart attack. In some patients coronary occlusion causes only mild pain, tightness or vague discomfort which may be ignored. The myocardium is however damaged.

oncology – The branch of medical science dealing with tumors, including the origin, development, diagnosis, and treatment of cancer.

open-heart surgery – Open-heart surgery is done while the bloodstream is diverted through a heart-lung machine. Some of the different types of open-heart surgeries are valve replacements, coronary bypass, and heart transplants.

P

pacemaker – A pacemaker is an electronic device used to treat patients who have symptoms caused by abnormally slow heartbeats. A pacemaker is capable of keeping track of the patient's heartbeats. If the patient's heart is beating too slowly, the pacemaker will generate electrical signals similar to the heart's natural signals, causing the heart to beat faster. The purpose of the pacemaker is to maintain heartbeats so that adequate oxygen and nutrients are delivered through the blood to the organs of the body.

pacemaker dependent – Heavily or totally dependent on a pacemaker to keep your heart beating.

pharmacological – The science dealing with the preparation, uses, and especially the effects of drugs.

Plaque – Plaque is a fatty material made up of cholesterol, calcium, and other substances in the blood. To understand why plaque is a problem, compare a healthy artery to an artery with atherosclerosis. A healthy artery is like a rubber tube. It is smooth and flexible, and blood flows through it freely. If the heart has to work harder, such as when a person exercises, a healthy artery can stretch to let more blood flow to the body's tissues. An artery with atherosclerosis is more like a clogged pipe. Plaque narrows the artery and makes it stiff. This limits the flow of blood to the tissues. When the heart has to work harder, the stiff arteries can't flex to let more blood through, and the tissues don't get enough blood and oxygen. (WebMD.com)

psychologist – A person trained and educated to perform psychological research, testing, and therapy. Psychologists study the physical, cognitive, emotional, and social aspects of behavior, and provide mental health care in hospitals, clinics, schools, and private practices.

physiologically – Being in accord with or characteristic of the normal functioning of a living organism.

PVC - Arrhythmias arising in the ventricle that are more likely to be found in people with more serious heart disease but may also be found in healthy individuals. Premature ventricular complex, or PVC: This electrical impulse starts in the ventricle causing the heart to beat earlier than expected. Usually, the heart returns to its normal rhythm right away.

R

restenosis – When an artery or stent will sometimes collapse or close off again.

rotablation – A nonsurgical technique for treating diseased arteries in which a special catheter with a diamond-coated tip is guided to the point of narrowing in the artery, spins at high speeds, and grinds away the blockage or plaque on the artery walls. It is not safe to rotablate a coronary vessel more then a few times.

S

stent – A small, expandable wire tube called a stent is often permanently inserted into the artery during angioplasty. A very thin guide wire is inside the catheter. The guide wire is used to move a balloon and the stent into the coronary artery. A balloon is placed inside the stent and inflated, which opens the stent and pushes it into place against the artery wall. The balloon is then deflated and removed, leaving the stent in place. Balloon angioplasty is the most common method of inserting stents, although sometimes stents are placed without the use of a balloon. Because the stent is mesh like, the cells lining the blood vessel grow through and around the stent to help secure it. (WebMD.com)

sternum – The sternum is a long, flat bone located in the center of the chest. It connects to the rib bones via cartilage, forming the rib cage with them, and thus helps to protect the lungs, heart, and major blood vessels from physical trauma. The sternum is sometimes cut open to gain access to the thoracic contents when performing cardiothoracic surgery.

stroke – A stroke, sometimes called a "brain attack," occurs when blood flow to an area in the brain is cut off. As a result, the brain cells, deprived of the oxygen and glucose needed to survive, die. If not caught early, permanent brain damage can result.

T

tachycardia – A rapid heart rate, usually defined as greater than 100 beats per minute.

U

underdeployed – A stent is not fully expanded, leaving a small "pocket" or space between the stent and the wall of the artery. This is dangerous as it can cause restenosis and movement in the artery.

V

VAD – A ventricular assist device (VAD) is a mechanical pump that helps a weakened heart pump blood throughout the body. It is used as a "bridge-to-transplant" for those who are hospitalized with heart failure and waiting for a donor heart to be available.

ENDNOTES

INTRODUCTION

[1] David Swartz. *Dancing with Broken Bones*. Illinois: David C. Cook Publishing Co., 1985. pg. 41.

CHAPTER ONE

[2] Bryan Duncan. "A Heart Like Mine." Love Takes Time, Myrrh, 1999

[3] Oswald Chambers. *My Utmost For His Highest*. Michigan: Discovery House Publishers, 1992, February 27.

[4] Jonel Aleccia. *The Spokesman Review* Spokane, WA February 14, 2007 March 2008 http://www.lcnw.org/info/news/pages/2007-02-14-wa.html

[5] ibid

[6] Dr. Mimi Guarneri M.D., FACC. *The Heart Speaks*. New York: Touchstone, 2007, pg. 158.

[7] John Eldridge. *Waking the Dead: The Glory of a Heart Fully Alive*. Tennessee: Thomas Nelson, Inc., 2003, pg. 39.

[8] Ilan Wittstein, M.D. Hopkins cardiologist. Johns Hopkins Medicine, February 9, 2005 April 2008 http://www.hopkinsmedicine.org/Press_releases/2005/02_10_05.html

CHAPTER TWO

[9] Lewis Carroll. *Alice's Adventures in Wonderland*. 1865

[10] University of Washington Television. January 2008 <http: //www.uwtv.org/newsletter/insider_1207.asp>)

[11] ibid

[12] November 2007, Public Citizen. <http://www.citizen.org/documents/FCT-Why_Doctors_Practice_Where_04-05-04.pdf>)

[13] Dr. Mimi Guarneri M.D., FACC. *The Heart Speaks*. New York: Touchstone, 2007

[14] Charles R. Swindoll. *Hope in Hurtful Times: A Study of 1 Peter*. California: Insight for Living, 1990, pg.

[15] ibid

[16] Tom Lutey. "She Needs a Christmas Miracle." *The Spokesman Review*, Spokane, WA, 12-8-2003, Tom Lutey, Exit 289

[17] Susan Gvozdas. "SHE'S TOO WELL." *Central Penn* Business Journal. Harrisburg, PA. March, 2004

[18] Thomas Stegmann Professor, M.D. "Article Being Submitted for Publication." May, 2008

[19] Joni Eareckson Tada. *Joni*. New York: Bantam, 1978

[20] Jill Briscoe. *Faith Enough to Finish*. Illinois: Tyndale House Publishers, 2001, pg. 170.

CHAPTER THREE

[21] Mark Farner. cond. audiocassette. "Isn't It Amazing." Just Another Injustice, Royal Tapestry Music, 1988

[22] Cindy Mah. "MAH'S MATTERS" Taken from a newsletter to her family. Her husband is battling stage 2 colon cancer. 2005

[23] Nicole E. Squibbs, Sun Staff Writer "Duck shot by arrow is recovering." Yuma Sun. Yuma, AZ, 19 May 2007 http: //www.yumasun.com/news/duck_34132___article.html/arrow_haugo.html

[24] Phillip Keller. *A Shepherd Looks at Psalm 23*. Michigan: Daybreak Books, 1970, pg. 90.

[25] Nick Vujicic. <http://www.lifewithoutlimbs.org> June 2008 Front Page

[26] ibid

[27] M.G., D.D. Easton, *Easton's 1897 Bible Dictionary*. Tennessee: Thomas Nelson

[28] David Wilkerson. *Times Square Church Pulpit Series*, June 13, 2005

[29] Tim Hansel. *You Gotta Keep Dancin': In the Midst of Life's Hurts, You Can Choose Joy!*. Illinois: David C. Cook Publishing, 1985, pg. 123.

CHAPTER FOUR

[30] Nancy Missler. *Private Worship: The Key to Joy*. Coeur d'Alene, Idaho: The King's High Way Ministries, 2002, pg. 49.

[31] Kenneth W. Osbeck. *Amazing Grace, 366 Inspiring Hymn Stories for Daily Devotions*. Grand Rapids, Michigan: Kregel Publications, 2002, pg. 261.

[32] Sermon Index.net, June 2008, http://www.sermonindex.net/modules/articles/index.php?view=article&aid=6023

[33] Lisa Bevere. *Out of Control and Loving it!.* Florida: Creation House, 1996, pg. 63.

[34] June 2008, < http://www.webmd.com/brain/tc/amyotrophic-lateral-sclerosis-als-topic-overview>

[35] David Swartz. *Dancing with Broken Bones*. Illinois: David C. Cook Publishing Co., 1985, pg. 41.

[36] Nancy Missler. "Faith in the Night Season, Remaining in His Presence," *Personal Update*, Koinonia House, October 2001

CHAPTER FIVE

[37] Larry Crabb. *Shattered Dreams.* Colorado: Waterbrook Press, 2001, pg. 165.

[38] Oswald Chambers. *My Utmost for His Highest*, January 29. Tennessee: Discovery House Publishers, 1992, January 29.

[39] Kenneth W. Osbeck. *101 More Hymn Stories*. Grand Rapids, Michigan: Kregel Publications, 1982, pg. 183.

[40] Nancy Missler. *The Choice*. Coeur d'Alene, Idaho: Koinonia House, 2001, pg. 71.

[41] Carolyn Custis James. *Lost Women of the Bible*: The *Women We Thought We Knew*. Michigan: Zondervan, 2008, pg. 94.

[42] ibid

[43] Larry Crabb. *Shattered Dreams.* Colorado: Waterbrook Press, 2001, pg. 94.

CHAPTER SIX

[44] "Give Your Body a Boost With Laughter." February 2008 http: //women.webmd.com/guide/give-your-body-boost-with-laughter

[45] "Humor, Laughter and Health: BRINGING MORE HUMOR AND LAUGHTER INTO OUR LIVES." http:// www.helpguide.org/life/humor_laughter_health.htm

[46] Tim Hansel. *You Gotta Keep Dancin': In the Midst of Life's Hurts, You Can Choose Joy!*. Illinois: David C. Cook Publishing, 1985, pg. 82.

CHAPTER SEVEN

[47] Kathleen Prentice. “When a Caregiver Needs Care.” *Heart Insight Magazine*. May 2008 < http://www.heartinsight.com/pt/re/wkhc/fulltext.01271221-200802000-00009.htm;jsessionid=LXnhVvpRhGHbzKVsd2GyXsdZfyLsMKrnN8vTN1nWvTw2vTy7vLGL!-1179726830!181195629!8091!-1>

[48] Joni Eareckson Tada. *Joni*. New York: Bantam, 1978

[49] Jeff Kuntz. “Hey You!” Email to author. 13 November 2003

[50] W. Hodding Carter.”Heroes, Most Valuable Player: *Reader's Digest*, May 2008

[51] Tim Hansel. *You Gotta Keep Dancin': In the Midst of Life's Hurts, You Can Choose Joy!*. Illinois: David C. Cook Publishing, 1985, pg. 66.

[52] Charles Siebert. “Carol Palumbo Waits for Her Heart.” *New York Times Magazine*, April 13, 1997

CHAPTER EIGHT

[53] “Bride dies during marriage's first dance.” AP news story. Sat Feb 9, 7:04 PM ET

[54] Francois de Fenelon. *The Seeking Heart*, The SeedSowers Christian Publishing House, 1993

CONCLUSION

[55] Charles R. Swindoll. *Hope in Hurtful Times: A Study of 1 Peter*. California: Insight for Living, 1990

[56] Mike Webb. An email to the author. February 2005

[57] Nancy DeMoss. Taken from *Revive Our Hearts* with is a ministry partnership of *Life Action Ministries*, *Back to the Bible* and *FamilyLife Today*. Daily Program Tuesday, November 26, 2002 March 2008 http://www.reviveourhearts.com/radio/today/23187

[58] David Wilkerson. "The Importance of Having the Peace of Christ." *Pulpit Series Newsletter*, November 13, 2006

Heart Disease and Organ Donation Information

43,000 women a year die from breast cancer, while 500,000 women die yearly from heart disease. Heart disease is still the number one killer of both men and women in the United States.

¤ ¤ ¤

"In December of 1967, a South African surgeon, Dr. Christiaan Barnard, transplanted the heart of a 23-year-old woman killed in a motor vehicle accident into the chest of a middle-aged man. He lived for eighteen days, until the powerful drugs used to suppress rejection weakened him and he died of pneumonia. The second patient to receive a heart transplant, at the hands of Dr. Adrian Kantrowitz in the United States, lived only six hours. But Dr. Barnard's next heart-transplant patient lived for 18 months and became a symbol of hope for victims of heart disease. All over the world patients were asking and receiving the new miracle operation.

"But this breakthrough has come with limitations, too. The problem with heart transplants now has become finding enough hearts. Today in the United States alone,

2 million people suffer from congestive heart failure. When drug treatments fail, transplants are the best hope. But less than 2,500 donor hearts are available each year, leaving thousands of patients desperate for an alternative." (NOVA Online, Pioneers of Heart Surgery, http://www.pbs.org/wgbh/nova/heart/pioneers.html)

¤ ¤ ¤

Biblical References Concerning Organ Donation:

What does the Bible say about organ translation and the decision to "Donate Life?

Genesis 2:21-23, "So the LORD God caused a deep sleep to fall upon the man, and he slept; then He took one of his ribs and closed up the flesh at that place. The LORD God fashioned into a woman the rib which He had taken from the man, and brought her to the man. The man said, this is now bone of my bones, and flesh of my flesh; she shall be called Woman, because she was taken out of Man."

¤ ¤ ¤

Deuteronomy 30:19 "I call heaven and earth to witness against you today, that I have set before you life and death, the blessing and the curse. So choose life in order that you may live, you and your descendants"

¤ ¤ ¤

Leviticus 19:18b "But you shall love your neighbor as yourself; I am the LORD."

Matthew 10:8 "Heal the sick, raise the dead, cleanse the lepers, cast out demons. Freely you received, freely give."

⌑ ⌑ ⌑

John 15:12,13 "This is My commandment, that you love one another, just as I have loved you. 'Greater love has no one than this that one lay down his life for his friends.'"

⌑ ⌑ ⌑

1 Corinthians 15:35,42,44,50 "But someone will say, 'How are the dead raised? And with what kind of body do they come?' So also is the resurrection of the dead It is sown a perishable body, it is raised an imperishable body; It is sown a natural body, it is raised a spiritual body. If there is a natural body, there is also a spiritual body. Now I say this, brethren, that flesh and blood cannot inherit the kingdom of God; nor does the perishable inherit the imperishable."

⌑ ⌑ ⌑

Judeo-Christian Facts about Organ Donation:

Jewish law proclaims the truth of the commandment in Leviticus 19:16: "Thou shall not stand idly by the blood of thy neighbor." The duty to save life supersedes any other law. One principle can be singled out for its prominence in Jewish bioethical discourse: the sanctity of human life and the duty to save and preserve it wherever possible.

"Giving oneself and one's possessions voluntarily for the wellbeing of others and without compulsion is a Christian duty." The Church of England, on organ donation.

¤ ¤ ¤

All major religions support organ and tissue donation and believe it's an act of human kindness.

¤ ¤ ¤

Death need not be the final comment of our lives. Instead of one stone marker at the head of our grave, there could be living memorials, real people with real families whose lives have been put back together through the gift of life. This is Christianity at it best: sharing one's own life for the purpose of helping someone else.

Risk factors you can control:
* High Blood Pressure
* Tobacco Smoke
* High Blood Cholesterol
* Physical Activity
* Obesity
* Diabetes

Risk factors you can't control:
* Increasing Age
* Sex (gender)
* Race
* Family Medical History
* Previous Heart Attack or Stroke

We have information to help you identify and manage your risk factors. Contact us and take the first step towards preventing a heart attack or stroke.

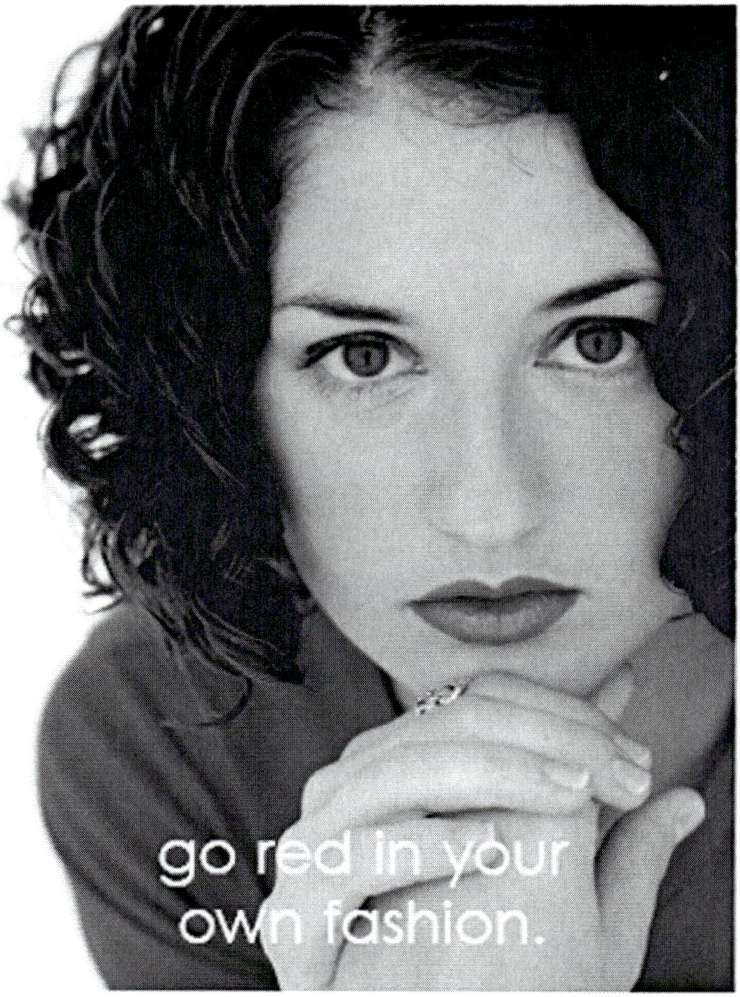

go red, anyway you want... eat red - **apples**, **cherries**, **tomatoes**, leave red **kisses** on someone's cheek. laugh so hard your **face** turns red. but whatever you do, do it for **your heart**. take a moment everyday and put your hand on your heart, and then make your own promise to be **heart healthy**.

Go Red for women

American Heart Association

Learn and Live

www.goredforwomen.org
1-888-MY HEART

American
Red Cross

Change a Life: Donate Blood!

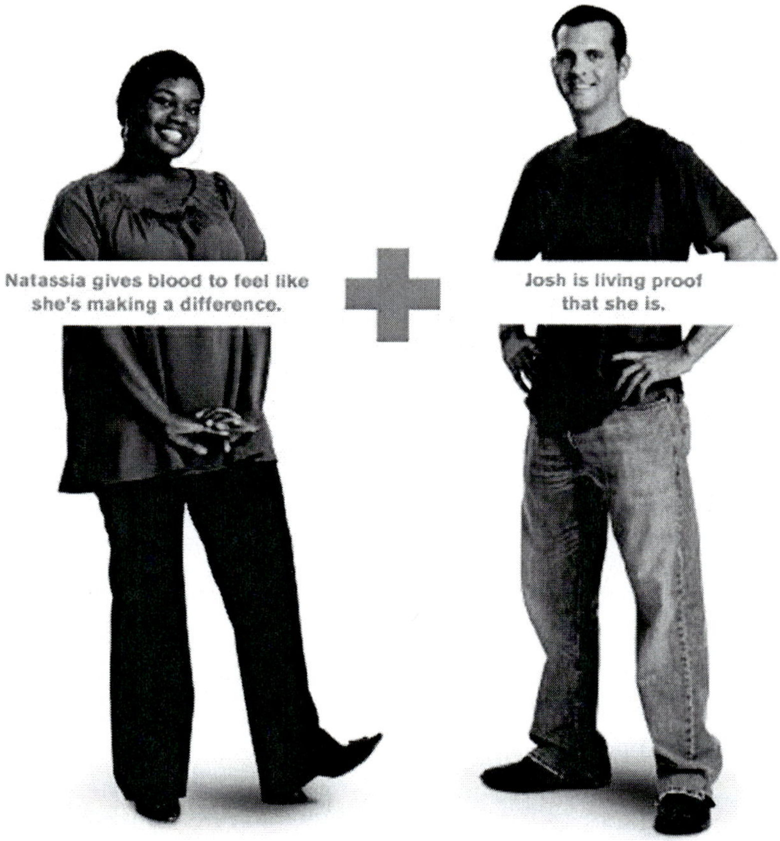

Donate blood today and change a life, starting with your own.
Call 1-800-GIVE LIFE or visit givelife.org.

American Red Cross

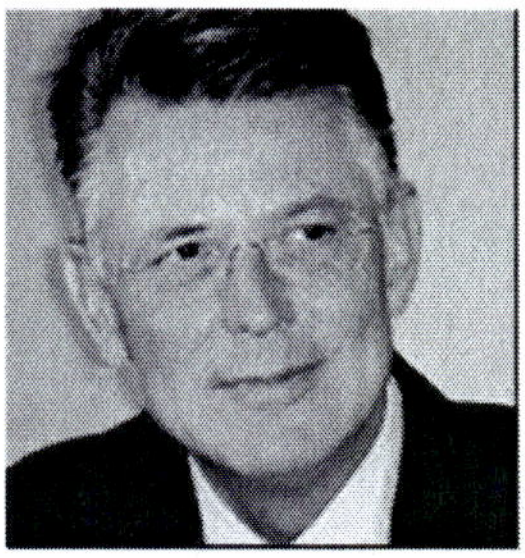

Thomas J. Stegmann, M.D., Ph.D.

CardioVascular
BioTherapeutics, Inc.

Dr. Thomas J. Stegmann's discovery of ways to stimulate growth of new blood vessels in the human heart opens up an exciting new area of biotechnology and medical treatment for cardiovascular disease. His research and subsequent trials have been articulated in an acclaimed volume, New Vessels for the Heart: Angiogenesis as New Treatment for Coronary Heart Disease: The Story of its Discovery and Development, published in 2005.

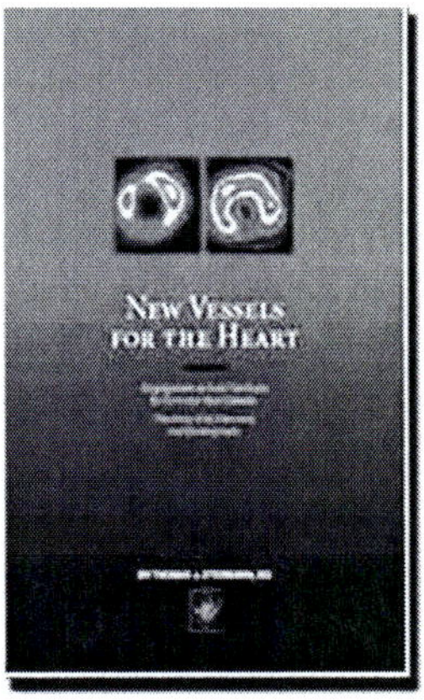

New Vessels for the Heart
by Thomas J. Stegmann, M.D., Ph.D.

This publication explains his discovery, the first scientific steps, and the 13-year journey that led to the current status of CVBT's human clinical trials in the United States. Dr. Stegmann describes the fascinating extension of that new treatment principle to represent an overwhelming potential for the therapy of a variety of diseases, such as stroke, wound-healing disturbances, chronic back pain, neurological disorders and others.

Now, you can read the story of the development and discovery of CVBT-141A for yourself in Dr. Stegmann's book.

Holding a Woman's Heart in My Hands
by Thomas J. Stegmann, M.D., Ph.D.

This informative booklet addresses the unique medical issues women's heart disease presents in both diagnosis and treatment, and how angiogenesis—the growth of new blood vessels in the heart—could be a new medical therapy to treat this disease, which kills more than 480, 000 women a year, according to the American Heart Association.

To request a complimentary copy of this booklet, please send an email with your name & mailing address to womensheartdisease@cvbt.com.

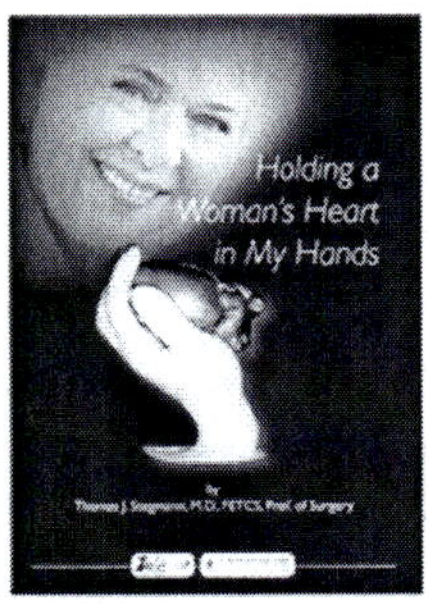

Visit CVBT's Website for more info

CardioVascular BioTherapeutics Inc.
1635 Village Center Circle, Suite 250
Las Vegas, Nevada 89134
www.cvbt.com